Anger, resentment and forgiveness:

How to get your inappropriate anger under reasonable control

By Dr Jim Byrne

With Renata Taylor-Byrne

Published by the Institute for E-CENT Publications, in cooperation with KDP-Amazon. 2019

Contents

Preface

The E-CENT theory of anger says that anger is one of our basic emotions. It's innate. It was selected by nature for its survival value. We would not survive for long without an innate sense of angering in response to abuse or neglect. We also would not survive for long if we did not quickly learn how to *moderate* our anger as young children. My anger is a two-edged sword. It can help to protect me, and it can attract hostile reactions from others.

My **basic** emotion of anger is elaborated into a *higher cognitive emotion* through modelling by my mother and father and significant others in the first few years of my life. And also through my successful and my unsuccessful experiences of engaging in conflict with others.

I may become an *exploder*, who erupts in the faces of others. I may become an *imploder*, who keeps his anger inside. Or I may hide my anger from myself (repress it) and then project it into my environment where it may frighten me.

So anger is a socialized emotion, and if you grew up with angry people, you are likely to be prone to angering yourself when provoked; or you might feel fearful of your own anger, or the anger of others.

~~~

Healthy anger is present-time defence of your legitimate rights in the face of inappropriate behaviour by another person. Healthy or *reasonable* anger is the fuel that drives our **assertive** behaviours. It pushes us to engage in *constructive conflict*, when that is *necessary*!

To ask for what you want, which is legitimately yours to request, requires a certain level of 'fire in your belly'. If you lack that fire (that *reasonable* level of anger), then you will tend to 'wimp-out'; to act passively and let other people control you, or intimidate you, or deny you your reasonable share of the social stage.

Unhealthy or *unreasonable* anger is an over-reaction to a frustrating or insulting stimulus from another person or external force. Unhealthy or unreasonable anger leads to **aggressive** actions and destructive conflict.

We teach the following eight insights to our anger management clients:

1. You were born with *an **innate capacity** to develop angry,* anxious and depressed responses to your social environment - in response to frustrations, threats and losses.

2. You then encountered your mother, who already had a 'style of relating', based on her attachment experience of her own mother and father. She would inevitably have shaped your emotional expression by:

(a) Modelling an approach to relationship and emotions; and:

(b) Rewarding and penalizing you for your daily emotion expressions, including your angry outbursts in the first couple of years of your life.

3. Your father's approach to relationship, including emotion expression, especially his way of expressing (or suppressing) anger, would have been the next major influence on the development of your emotion expression, including your way of being angry - implosive or explosive; appropriate or inappropriate.

4. If both of your parents had a secure attachment to their own parents, they would have had a warm but assertive approach to relating to you. From them you would have learned to be secure in your relationship with them, and, by extension, in virtually all subsequent people-encounters. You would have learned to express healthy or appropriate anger in an *assertive* way - to ask for what you want, and to say no to what you do not want. You would not have any significant problems with anger.

5. However, if one or both of your parents had an insecure attachment to their own parents, they would have had an insecure attachment to you, and been either explosively or implosively angry with you when you frustrated them or broke their personal rules. From them, you would have learned to engage in unhealthy or inappropriate anger expression of an explosive or implosive type, or a mixture of the two, varying from situation to situation. (Or you might have learned to be *passive* in those situations in which you felt frightened or fearful of reprisals, but *aggressive* in those situations where you felt no constraint of fearfulness!)

6. If you want to change your relationship style today, you need to experience secure relationship with another person - possibly a romantic partner, or a good therapist who understands how to build a secure

relationship with you. You need to learn the difference between *appropriate* and *inappropriate* anger. And also that **explosive** anger - (like shouting and using aggressive body language) - costs you, in terms of damage to relationships and careers, for examples; and that implosive anger - (like sulking and stewing in your own angry juices, or withdrawing aggressively) - damages your ongoing happiness, your relationships at home and at work, and ultimately your physical and mental health.

7. You can improve your relationship and attachment style by studying and applying new ideas from emotional literacy and self-assertion. And I can teach those ideas and skills to you.

8. But you are also a body-mind, and so your approach to managing your diet, physical exercise, self-talk (inner dialogue), and relaxation/ meditation are also important. And it is easier to develop a secure attachment style if your romantic partner is already secure.

9. See Appendix A for specific dietary guidance and advice. And see also Section E12 of Appendix E.

~~~

When an E-CENT counsellor works with an angry client, they may work on

- deep, emotional and attachment issues from early childhood; or on

- present-time assertiveness skills,

- and/or advice on important dietary changes,

- and/or recommendations regarding regular physical exercise,

- plus consideration of sleep hygiene issues,

- and/or teaching the client how to reframe their anger-inducing experiences,

- and/or changing some elements of their philosophy of life (as they show up in their inner dialogues about anger-inducing situations)

– and/or to change some (controllable) aspect of their social or physical environment with which they have been putting up!

~~~

Managing anger with diet and nutrition

In Part 1 of our book on diet and nutrition, Renata Taylor-Byrne (2017) explored - among other things - the key ways in which *diet can influence anger*. Some of the key findings were as follows:

Firstly, (unlike in the case of depression) there is at least one study which supports the idea that there is a link between low serotonin levels and the expression of anger, annoyance and irritation (specifically, low serotonin was linked to a reduced ability to self-manage rising levels of anger). She also presents evidence which showed that 5HTP, a natural nutritional supplement (from a West African medicinal plant called *Griffonia simpicifolia*), can be effective in restoring serotonin, an important neurotransmitter within the brain, thus reducing the expression of angry and hostile behaviour, as evidenced by Julie Ross's (2002) case study example.

The levels of copper and manganese in the client's body can have an effect on levels of anger; and the link between violent offenders (in prison) and the condition known as 'reactive hypoglycaemia' (where blood sugar levels fall to low after eating high carbohydrate meals) has been established, by research which has been conducted into extremely aggressive behaviour. This points to the need to investigate further the connection between fluctuating blood sugar levels and anger management problems.

Research has also established a definite link between a reduction in the consumption of sugar and refined foods, (on the one hand), and anger and anti-social behaviour, (on the other). In a similar vein, reductions in diets containing trans-fats, mainly involving hydrogenated fats in processed foods, led to a reduction in impatience, irritability and aggression in research participants.

Conversely, the link between pro-social behaviour and a healthy diet has also been evidenced by research. Dietary changes which increase the nutritional content of people's diets result in improvements in pro-social behaviour, and better emotion and mood control.

Finally, anger levels declined in prisoners whose diet has been supplemented with fish oils, vitamins and minerals: and it has been shown that omega 3 fats have a rapid and significant impact on aggression in children and adults.

For further information, please see Appendix E for specific dietary guidance and advice.

How anger can be reduced by exercise:

According to the British National Health Service website, anger is effectively reduced in intensity by exercising, including walking, swimming and yoga. Research studies have supported this view, and here are some examples which have provided valuable evidence in the role of exercise and anger reduction:

Research conducted by Joseph Tkacz, *et al.*, (2008), found that aerobic exercise regimes reduced anger expression among obese children. It was the first study which had been conducted to assess the value of having structured aerobic exercise sessions for overweight children, and the findings pointed to the value of exercise sessions after school.

Also, there was a study which investigated levels of anger amongst undergraduates at the University of Georgia. It was entitled: "Phys Ed: Can Exercise Moderate Anger?"(Reynolds, G., 2010) and was reported in the New York Times magazine. The 16 students selected were regularly oversensitive and their anger was easily triggered. After experiencing different research conditions designed to arouse their anger, and experienced firstly without the benefits of exercise, and then after they *had* exercised, it was apparent that there was a change in their levels of anger linked to the exercise program.

After the exercise they were able to show composure and self-assurance in the face of emotional provocation. The results of this experiment did reduce their levels of anger, prompting the lead researcher, Nathaniel Thoms, a stress physiologist, to say:

"Exercise, even a single bout of it, can have a robust prophylactic (therapeutic) effect against the build-up of anger…it's like taking an aspirin to combat heart disease. You reduce your risk".

This result is echoed by the advice of the Mayo Clinic Staff, who have written that the higher the levels of stress a person is experiencing, the more likely they are to have high levels of anger, and that these effects can be diminished by vigorous and pleasurable exercise.

For further information, please see Appendix F for more specific information on research into different forms of exercise.

~~~

Dealing with the deep roots of anger in childhood

According to Fisher (2005, page 158) much of the emotional pain that drives inappropriate, aggressive anger "...is connected to early traumatic experience". Childhood trauma can cause us to 'act out' (the old, incomplete, dramas) in the present moment, with the wrong people!

"Whenever there is a disproportionate amount of anger in response to an event, it is more than likely that unprocessed traumatic experiences from the past are manifesting themselves in the present". (Fisher, 2005, pages 159-160).

Fisher recommends working through the 'trauma cycle' with a trauma counsellor to overcome childhood distress that is driving current aggressive anger problems.

Lindenfield (2000) has a chapter about dealing with the backlog of unresolved anger. She points out that early childhood wounds may be inaccessible to you because:

(1)   You have (consciously) forgotten the pain, because you repressed it in order to cope with the hurt and get on with your life.

(2)   You might not think you have the right to feel wounded by hurtful experiences.

Gael Lindenfield's own childhood experience included having an alcoholic mother "...who lied, cheated and irresponsibly neglected and abandoned her children in order to indulge her own needs and wants". (Page 94).

If you have a backlog of unresolved anger from your childhood, adolescence or young adulthood, you can process that by keeping an anger management journal; attending an anger management group; or seeing an anger management counsellor.

In your anger management journal, write about anger problems in the present moment, and what they could be related to in your past. (See Byrne, 2009a[1]; and Byrne, 2010a[2]).

Write the story of your childhood, and try to describe what happened to you – or did not happen to you, which should have happened – which was clearly unfair, unreasonable, or hurtful. Visualize yourself going back and confronting those situations. Write of yourself as if speaking to the people who treated you badly. Assert your reasonable rights with them. Take your journal to a counsellor, and talk through your issues.

For more on resolving childhood sources of anger, by completing your experience in the here-and-now, see Appendix D.

~~~

Dr Jim Byrne, Doctor of Counselling

Hebden Bridge, March 2019

~~~

Part 1: A quick introduction to anger management principles

In Part 1 of this book, you will find three chapters.

Chapter 1 will introduce you to ten core principles of the system of anger management that I teach to my counselling and therapy clients.

This system recognizes that human beings have bodies as well as minds; that their emotions are shaped in their family of origin; and that they are always connected to a current social environment (including family, friends, neighbours, work colleagues, and perhaps a romantic partner).

Because of this multi-dimensional nature of being human, we have to deal with everything that affects the body-brain-mind of the angry individual.

However, we cannot teach everything all at once, so we begin with the ten most important principles; and then gradually add the other dimension later.

In Chapter 2, I explore the question of how to forgive others, and why you should forgive others, for their transgressions against you. Forgiveness is the royal road out of the suffering of ongoing anger.

And finally, in Chapter 3, I present my own Six Windows Model, which teaches six ways to re-think or *re-frame* your anger-inducing problems, so that you no longer have to be painfully angry when things go wrong in your life. By changing the way you perceive difficult situations, you get a new set of emotional and behavioural responses. You learn to calm yourself down *despite* the difficulties you face.

~~~

Get your anger under reasonable control

Chapter 1: Ten Principles of Anger Management Counselling

By Dr Jim Byrne

Copyright (c) Jim Byrne: 2014 –2019

Introduction

Anger is one of the main emotions that humans feel in certain kinds of stressful situations. The other two are anxiety and depression.

Anger is the emotion that corresponds to the 'fight response' when an animal or human feels threatened, or (in the case of humans), seriously frustrated by another person, or insulted by somebody, or confronted by the bad behaviour of others.

In civilized societies, anger can be either *appropriate* to the circumstances surrounding the angry individual; or *excessive* and *aggressive*. (Or sometimes, as with passive individuals, their anger may be *lacking*, and too *weak*!)

In order to teach our clients how to manage their anger appropriately, we have evolved a set of principles which can help to summarize coping self-talk, and coping actions.

Here are the first ten such principles:

Principle 1: Anger is natural, normal and innate, or inborn into each of us. So you should not try to get rid of *all traces* of your anger.

Anger can keep us safe in a dangerous world. But it can also lead us to engage in conflict that is *against our best interests*; and harmful to others (which is at least immoral, and sometimes illegal!) (So anger can be constructive or destructive).

Anger can help us to know when we are being threatened, exploited or exposed to danger, and help us to fight our way out. And it is good to learn a system of self-defence which will reduce your aggression, and keep your powder dry until you absolutely have to use it!

It is often the case that what is required is a *moderate level of anger*, directed in the form of assertive actions or assertive communications (which are not aggressive or hostile or harmful or hurtful of others).

~~~

Principle 2: Because anger is natural and normal, that does not justify anybody discharging their anger in an ***unthinking*** or ***uncontrolled*** way. Just as the elimination of waste products from the body is natural and normal, and that we have ***socialized ways*** of doing that decorously - (meaning, politely and with restraint) - so also do civilized individuals have decorous (or polite and restrained) ways of managing their anger.

Furthermore, in a family that knows how to manage its emotions well, the children learn to control their anger so that they feel reasonable levels of anger, and avoid excessive, destructive anger.

If your family did not teach you to control your anger to reasonable, assertive levels – and to avoid aggressive and destructive anger outbursts; and to avoid passive 'wimping out' – you can still learn how to do that *today*. It is never too late to learn new approaches to emotional self-management.

~~~

Principle 3: An angry reaction to frustration or insult is a manifestation of the **fight response** which is innate in all animals. But you cannot fight a traffic jam, or too many emails, or a clever insult; or even a sense of being neglected. Therefore, you have to rewire yourself to respond with something other than anger in those situations where anger will not guide you into the right course of action. The first piece of rewiring that you could benefit from is this:

Teach yourself, over and over again, to accept the things you <u>cannot</u> change and to only try to change the things which are fairly clearly <u>changeable</u>.

For example, remember that we can (often – with much difficulty!) change aspects of our selves (some of our behaviours, values, beliefs, etcetera). But we cannot reliably change other people; and certainly not often; or routinely. But we do have the right to try to influence our partners and significant others, to the degree that we allow them to influence us. So use influencing strategies instead of anger to try to change your partner or a significant other.

And teach yourself to *laugh off insults and affronts!* This will rob your adversaries of the victory of seeing how much they have upset you!

~~~

Principle 4: Anger is very often a 'false friend'.

In a life threatening situation, you have to act first and think later. But most of the situations in which you become angry are (most likely) far from being life threatening!

Inappropriate anger whispers in your ear that you are right and the other person is wrong; that you are being taken advantage of or abused; and that the other person must be punished for this transgression. Very often, *this is not the only way to look at the situation*. And this is often *a false statement!*

The other person may be *unaware* of the fact that they are causing you a problem. And/or: The problem they are causing you may be of a kind that you also, in your turn, *unavoidably* cause to other people – and you would not want them to get angry with you for this act.

So don't automatically trust *the voice of anger-inducement* in your ear. Challenge it. Ask yourself:

Is this true?

Is there a better way of looking at the situation?

*Will getting angry really **help me** in any significant way?*

Or will it actually make matters worse?

~~~

Principle 5: *Inappropriate anger* is like picking up a hot coal with the intention of throwing it at the person who insulted or frustrated you, or broke your personal rules.

When you pick up that hot coal, **you** are the one who gets burned; just as, when you swallow *the poison of resentment*, **you** are the one who is going to be made ill by it. The person you resent or hate is not going to die because of your resentment or hatred.

5.

Resentment *attaches us* to the resented person.

Hatred *attaches us* to the hated person.

We get **stuck** to those people and situations against which we respond angrily.

Instead of picking up a hot coal to throw at those who seem to rile us, we need to learn to *respond appropriately*. And **sometimes**, responding appropriately means *doing nothing!* Letting it go! (One way to do this is to persuade yourself that, very often, the 'winning formula' is to accept that *life will frustrate and harry you* – but you have **the power** to let that wash over you, and not to get stuck!)

At other times, responding appropriately might mean using a well thought out **assertive** communication message. (Such as: "I am *angry* that you did [X], because it has [negative effect Y] on my life. And I would *prefer it* if you would not do that again!" Or: "I am angry that you would not do Y for me; and I really think it was unfair, given what I do for you!"

(Search for online information on how to assert yourself).

~~~

Principle 6: Avoid developing automatic, habitual anger triggers – because some situations that look like they justify anger actually do no such thing. You may often feel affronted in situations where no affront exists and nothing needs to be done by you. Some contexts in which doing nothing is called for – in which case you should let it go - include:

(1) _Situations of **chaos**_, in which **nobody** could be expected to have prevented the frustration or difficulty – for example, a busy motorway (Highway, autobahn), or a crowded pavement, and somebody 'gets in your way!'

(2) _Lack of **intent** to offend_ on the part of the offending party. Imagine you are boating on a foggy river. I big white boat comes out of the fog. It is heading straight towards your boat, and likely to cause a collision and some damage to your hull. You become very angry. Then you notice that the boat has nobody on board – it is adrift!

Many people are just like that boat. Nobody (conscious) is on board! Non-consciousness abounds. Humans are creatures of habit! Do not assume *intentional* *offence* as your default position.

~~~

Principle 7: Distinguish between what you can control and what you cannot control.

If you **can** *control* some frustration or insult, or unfairness, or the offending behaviour of another person, then you should *take appropriate action* to do that; (unless you decide that it is not important enough to justify the energy you would have to expend to control or change it – in which case you should accept it or laugh it off.)

If you **cannot** *control* some frustration or insult, or bad behaviour of another person, then *you must come to terms with it* – and **accept** it – if you are to avoid angering yourself *unnecessarily* and to no good end!

Teach yourself this mantra: "I accept the things I cannot change, and only try to change the things I think I probably can". Repeat this mantra several times every morning and evening, until it becomes part of your core philosophy of life.

~~~

Principle 8: Distinguish between passive, aggressive and assertive options. (*Inappropriate anger* means always going for the *aggressive* option). See Appendix C, and also aspects of Appendix B.

Sometimes an individual may put up with a lot of injustice, unfairness, or frustration, or insults: and then, finally, they flip over into rageful anger. This is often called 'the passive-aggressive modality'. The individual is *too passive for too long*, and then they become *too aggressive*.

In Transactional Analysis (TA), the passive phase is called "Collecting Brown Stamps" – because the passive-aggressive individual is collecting a stamp (or record of offence; or a record of a negative experience) each time they are offended against; and one day they intend (consciously or non-consciously) *to cash in their book of stamps* (when it is 'full') for *an explosive outburst of aggressive anger*.

The passive-aggressive individual flips from passivity to aggression, and does not have a middle gear – just top and bottom: too little or too much.

Passive-aggressive behaviour can also involve an individual who is angry, but who operates indirectly, covertly; and denies that they are angry; but they put an 'untraceable spanner' in the works of those people with whom they are angry. (These people often engage in sabotage of others).

The passive-aggressive flip, and the indirect passive-aggression approach, are both unhelpful, destructive in the longer term, and counter-productive. They will not get you what you want – if what you want is better human relations, and a chance to get more of your wishes granted.

The solution to both of these passive-aggressive approaches is to *learn to be assertive*; which means: asking for what you want, and saying 'no' to what you do not want – and doing it in a non-aggressive manner.

~~~

Principle 9: In Rational Emotive therapy, the main target for anger-reduction is this:

Give up **demanding** that you ABSOLUTELY must not be frustrated, insulted or wronged.

It may often, or even normally, be the case that *you MORALLY should not* have to face particular forms of frustration by others; and you certainly should not be insulted by them, or wronged by them.

But we live in a world of *imperfect* fellow humans, and each of us has a **good** side and a **bad** side. So, as Marcus Aurelius used to teach, you should tell yourself each morning:

"Today I am going to run into all kinds of difficult, offensive, challenging, frustrating, insulting, malicious, untrustworthy and overbearing individuals. All of these states have been visited upon them because they (often) lack clarity about the nature of real Good and Evil!"

If you are thus forewarned; forearmed; you will not be surprised when a sleep-deprived individual - who still has too much alcohol washing around in their brain; and who had a big conflict with their partner before leaving home – pops up in front of you in a way that frustrates or insults you.

Let it go! You already knew you would run into him or her! Do you want to demonstrate that you are just as stupid, uncivilized and evil as they are proving to be?

~~~

Principle 10: In your intimate relationships it is important to maintain a 5:1 ratio of positive to negative moments. Therefore, you cannot resort to anger very often, and most often you will have to learn how to be *reasonably assertive*, instead of either passive or aggressive.

You must learn how to communicate and negotiate, instead of blustering and browbeating; or shouting and name-calling; all of which is aggressive and offensive, and damaging to your relationships.

Also, in close relationships, you should remember Dale Carnegie's rule: *Do not kick over the beehive, if you want to collect honey. If you offend your nearest and dearest, they will resent that, hold it against you, and you will not 'collect any honey' from them!*

~~~

Outside of intimate relationships, you might even need to maintain a 6:1 ratio of positive to negative moments, because work colleagues and other people are *less likely to make allowances for you*, in the way that a love partner often does!

So you have to learn how to get off it with people who frustrate you and break your personal rules. That can be seen as a straight choice:

- Get 'stuck on it' (in a state of anger) with significant others; or:

- 'Get off it' (*dump* or *defuse* the anger) for the sake of the relationship.

But do not try to 'swallow' the anger. That will not work. You will simply find that you have unwittingly 'collected a brown stamp'. (See Principle 8 above).

Instead, in order to 'get off it' with significant others - or even with strangers who frustrate you in public - you must learn to "forgive them their trespasses!" And that means "making it okay" that they did what they did; or failed to do what you wanted them to do. And "making it okay" very often results from *understanding why they did what they did*. It is often said that, "to understand all is to forgive all". (But do not become a masochist. If you are in a relationship with an angry person, and you cannot seem to defuse the situation, then you should get out for the sake of your dignity, and to enforce your right to be treated with respect as an equal human being!)

Forgiveness is the subject of Chapter 2, below.

~~~

Postscript: The major oversight in presenting these ten principles is this: Anger can be caused by eating foods high in trans-fats; or drinking alcohol; or eating a diet high in sugary foods. It can also be triggered by having insufficient sleep on a nightly basis, or even occasionally. And anger is difficult to sustain if you are: well rested; well exercised; in a harmonious relationship; and you eat little or no trans-fats; keep your alcohol and caffeine consumption low; and you get a good supply of omega-3 fatty acids, from oily fish, like salmon and sardines.

These aspects of anger-management are explored further in Part 4: Dr Jim's Stress and Anxiety Diet; and there is an Appendix (A) on the links between diet, exercise and sleep, on the one hand, and anger on the other.

~~~

Learning tip:

If you want change your behaviour – to become less angry – it is not going to be enough to simply read this chapter, or this whole book. If that is all you do, then the material you have read will quickly drain from your memory banks. In order to learn this material reliably, so you have it 'at your fingertips' when you run into an anger-inducing situation, you have got to re-read, and re-read this material, over and over again. To begin with, I recommend that you:

- *Mark* those sections that are most important to you personally - (perhaps with margin notes, or coloured pens) - knowing what your anger triggers tend to be.

- *Underline particular sentences* that are most helpful to you.

- Read this chapter *three times*:

      ❐ First reading completed.

      ❐ Second reading completed.

      ❐ Third reading completed.

And then:

- Revisit it weekly for a month:

> ❐ Firstly weekly revisit of this chapter (especially the bits you have marked and underlined!)

> ❐ Second weekly revisit of this chapter

> ❐ Third weekly revisit of this chapter

> ❐ Fourth weekly revisit of this chapter (especially the bits you have marked and underlined!)

- Then monthly for a year,

> ❐ ❐ ❐ ❐ ❐ ❐ ❐ ❐ ❐ ❐ ❐ ❐

- And then annually for five years.

> ❐ ❐ ❐ ❐ ❐

~~~

Get your anger under reasonable control

Chapter 2: Some thoughts on the subject of forgiveness

By Jim Byrne, Copyright © Jim Byrne, 2019

~~~

2.1. Introduction

> *"When a deep injury is done to us, we never recover until we forgive".*
>
> Alan Paton (South African writer)[3].

~~~

When we get stuck in a protracted or prolonged state of anger towards another person, we mainly harm ourselves. We harm our guts and our arteries and our hearts. And we destroy our own peace of mind.

Sometimes the solution is to assert our rights with the other person, and to get them to change. And then we can let go of the anger.

Sometimes we can reframe (or re-think or re-interpret) their offence, so that it no longer seems so bad; and the anger falls away.

But at other times, nothing will work except *to forgive them* their offence against us, so we can return to feeling at peace. (This does not mean that we forget what they did; nor does it mean that we will become reconciled with them. What it means is that we 'get off it' with them, so we can be at peace!)

In this chapter, I will:

1. Define forgiveness, using a range of dictionaries: of English, psychology, quotations, and philosophy; plus some major research studies;

2. Explore the nature of human anger, resentment and aggressive responses to transgressions by others; in the context of what we can control, and what we may or may not be able to influence;

3. Look briefly at character strengths, as the essential context for the development of forgiveness;

4. Sketch some elements of the art of forgiveness; and:

5. Present two process models of forgiveness:

> (a) One *general* model (which can be used by *anybody*, including individuals who are getting out of a couple relationship in which there is resentment on their side); and:

> (b) One for couples who want to *continue* in an ongoing relationship.

~~~

2.2. Forgiveness, anger and character

(a) Defining forgiveness

> *"It is easier to forgive an enemy than to forgive a friend".*
>
>> William Blake. (English poet). From Ratcliffe (2010), page 197.

~~~

The reason that it's harder to forgive a friend is that we expect to be treated well by our friends, and when they treat us badly, we feel particularly aggrieved.

According to my Oxford English dictionary, forgiveness means, not surprisingly, 'the act of forgiving'. And to 'Forgive' is defined like this:

> "Verb: 1. Stop feeling angry or resentful towards (someone) for an offence or mistake. 2. Excuse (an offence, flaw or mistake)."[4]

My dictionary of psychology[5], surprisingly, does *not* have a definition of forgiveness. However, some modern psychologists do work with the concept of 'forgiveness', and present their understanding of the meaning of the concept in their writings. Here is an example from a blog post at *Psychology Today* online:

> "Although there are a variety of definitions of forgiveness, research has suggested they all have 3 common components:

> 1. Gaining a more balanced view of the offender and the event

> 2. Decreasing negative feelings towards the offender and potentially increasing compassion

> 3. Giving up the right to punish the offender further or to demand restitution".

(Rubin Khoddam PhD, on the science of forgiveness)[6].

~~~

According to a research paper by the American Psychological Association (APA, 2006), forgiveness is defined as follows:

> "Forgiveness is a process (or the result of a process) that involves a change in emotion and attitude regarding an offender. Most scholars view this as an intentional and voluntary process, driven by a deliberate decision to forgive (...). This process results in decreased motivation to retaliate or to maintain estrangement from an offender despite their actions, and requires letting go of negative emotions toward the offender."[7]

According to Ben Dean (2005)[8]: "Baskin and Enright (2005, p. 80) distinguish forgiveness from condoning, excusing, reconciling, and forgetting".[9]

(b) The benefits of forgiveness

When we forgive somebody for a transgression against us, we become more peaceful and compassionate towards the offender. We no longer avoid them or act out our anger towards them. But this does not involve *forgetting* the transgression, or condoning or excusing it, but we may remember it in a *reformed* or *revised* way - a more *understanding* way. ("To understand all is to forgive all!")

What other *benefits* accrue from forgiving those who transgress against us? According to APA (2016), benefits include the fact that:

Forgiveness promotes psychological healing through positive changes in emotional states.

It also improves physical and mental health.

When we forgive others, this action helps to restore our sense of personal power.

And it helps "...to bring about reconciliation between the offended and offender". (However, reconciliation is *not* an *essential* feature of forgiveness as such. It is possible for one person to forgive another unilaterally, without any reconciliation, and still there will be the benefit of peace and psychological healing for the forgiving individual!)

~~~

(c) For and against forgiveness

My dictionary of philosophy[10] suggests that there are philosophical problems with the concept of forgiveness, the main one being that to forgive somebody for some harm or wrong they have done is to treat them *better than they deserve*. Although this might make sense in a system of perfect justice, humans and our social systems are *all imperfect*, and we often behave in a utilitarian fashion, where we pursue the 'greater good of the greater number', rather than perfect justice or perfect fairness.

On the other hand, as mentioned briefly above, people often do bad things for reasons which are *beyond their control* – such as the *habits* they acquired from the ways in which they were raised by their parents.

Longfellow said this more poetically when he wrote:

"If we could read the secret history of our enemies, we should see sorrow and suffering enough to disarm all hostility". (Page 32, Kornfield, 2002).

Long-term self-interest also can be used to justify forgiving somebody, even though this seems to involve treating them better than they deserve to be treated, given their bad treatment of the forgiving party. This can be illustrated by the following quotation by Thomas Fuller:

"(The person) (who) cannot forgive others breaks the bridge over which (they) must pass ..., for every person has need to be forgiven (at some point in time)".

And this principle was stated in reverse by Bill Clinton, the former US President, when he said:

"I believe any person who asks for forgiveness has to be prepared to give it"[11].

So, if I treat you better than you deserve to be treated, considering how badly you have treated me, my hope is that, further down the line, when I need to be forgiven by you or somebody else, for some transgression of mine, I can hope to be forgiven if I live in a world of pragmatic utilitarianism, and not in a world of *perfect or retributive justice*.

Furthermore, if you insist upon living in a world of perfect justice, of retributive justice, then how will you forgive yourself when you transgress your own moral rules, at various (unavoidable) points in the future of your (imperfect) life? If you will not forgive me my sins against you, how are you ever going to forgive yourself your own sins against your own moral code? And once you learn to forgive yourself, because your bad actions were caused by your own painful life's experiences, don't you then have to forgive others for their bad actions, which were driven by their painful life experiences?

~~~

(d) Understanding our negative responses to transgressions

When somebody offends us, or insults us, or frustrates or neglects us, we often feel angry and resentful. If we did not feel any resentment at all, we would be very vulnerable to being exploited and oppressed. Our angry reactions, *up to a certain point*, are constructive, and evolved naturally to enhance our survival.

The animals that arose through the millions of years of evolution of life on earth, which did not respond angrily or self-protectively, when threatened, died out, and did not live to reproduce.

We are the descendants of particular lines of evolving animals which were *sufficiently aggressive* to be able to defend themselves against attack, oppression and exploitation; but also *sufficiently cooperative and trusting* to be able to form communities. Communal living afforded us greater survival chances than isolated or solitary living.

In this sense, there is healthy (assertive) anger, and unhealthy (aggressive) anger; and also unhealthy passivity (or acquiescence in our own oppression) and healthy adaptability (or reasonable conformity to social norms).

(e) What we can and cannot control

When we are frustrated in our goals with other people; or we are insulted by their words or deeds; or neglected and treated unfairly by them; we have to ask ourselves:

> *"About this situation, what can I control, and what is beyond my control?"*

Once we have identified what we can control (in theory) we should, logically set out to try to control that event or object. If it turns out that we were wrong about being able to control it, after several serious attempts to control it, we might have to abandon our attempts to control it, and submit to its inevitability.

One of the things I have learned over the years is this: I can try to *influence* other people, and sometimes I am *successful* and sometimes I am *unsuccessful*. But I certainly cannot *control* them, nor should I even *try* to control them, because *controlling them* seems to me to imply that I interfere with their autonomy.

Of course, if some of their behaviours are a threat to my legitimate interests and needs, then I have the right to defend myself. I do this by having strong boundaries, which allow good things in, but endeavour strongly to keep bad things out. And my ultimate boundary in an intimate relationship, with a partner who shows an indifference to harming me, is to *leave*, and *never* return!

On the other hand, I have a better chance of controlling myself, some but not all of the time, in certain respects. Because I am a creature of habit (just like you!) I often fail to control myself, and when I do succeed in controlling myself, it is most often the result of strenuous efforts to do so!

So where does forgiveness fit into the picture?

(f) Character strengths

Each of us has a set of character strengths, derived from our early socialization by our parents, our wider family relationships, and our schooling[12]. Those character strengths can, and often do, include the virtue of forgiveness. Here is one comprehensive list of character strengths, from the discipline of Positive Psychology. Each of us will have some elements of these lists as developed or underdeveloped traits:

> ### The Virtue of Wisdom
>
> *Creativity: Original; adaptive; ingenuity*
>
> *Curiosity: Interest; novelty-seeking; exploration; openness to experience*
>
> *Judgment: Critical thinking; thinking things through; open-minded*
>
> *Love of Learning: Mastering new skills & topics; systematically adding to knowledge*
>
> *Perspective: Wisdom; providing wise counsel; taking the big picture view*
>
> ~~~

The Virtue of Courage

Bravery: Valour; not shrinking from fear; speaking up for what's right

Perseverance: Persistence; industry; finishing what one starts

Honesty: Authenticity; integrity

Zest: Vitality; enthusiasm; vigour; energy; feeling alive and activated

~~~

The Virtue of Humanity

Love: Both loving and being loved; valuing close relations with others

Kindness: Generosity; nurturance; care; compassion; altruism; "niceness"

Social Intelligence: Aware of the motives/feelings of oneself & others

~~~

The Virtue of Justice

Teamwork: Citizenship; social responsibility; loyalty

Fairness: Just; not letting feelings bias decisions about others

Leadership: Organizing group activities; encouraging a group to get things done

~~~

The Virtue of Temperance

Forgiveness: Mercy; accepting others' shortcomings; giving people a second chance

Humility: Modesty; letting one's accomplishments speak for themselves

Prudence: Careful; cautious; not taking undue risks

Self-Regulation: Self-control; disciplined; managing impulses & emotions

~~~

The Virtue of Transcendence

Appreciation of Beauty and Excellence: Awe; wonder; elevation

Gratitude: Thankful for the good; expressing thanks; feeling blessed

Hope: Optimism; future-mindedness; future orientation

Humour: Playfulness; bringing smiles to others; light-hearted

Spirituality: Religiousness; faith; purpose; meaning

~~~

So, forgiveness is one of our *twenty-four* **potential** *virtues.* But not all of us have all of those virtues in a developed form. If you want to find out which virtues you have developed more than others, then you can take a test here: The Via Institute on Character, here: https://www.viacharacter .org /www/ Character-Strengths-Survey

~~~

(g) To forgive or to hold a grudge?

> *"The stupid neither forgive nor forget; the naïve forgive and forget; the wise forgive but do not forget".*
>
> Thomas Szasz (Hungarian-born psychiatrist). From Ratcliffe (2010), page 198.

However, even before you set out to take that test, you will have a good idea whether or not you are likely to score highly or more modestly for the virtue of forgiveness.

Do you hold grudges? For how long? Do you feel resentment for long periods of time? Do you seek to inflict punishment on those who transgress against you?

If you have difficulty letting go of grudges and resentments; and you easily get stuck in resentment and alienation towards others, you could benefit from thinking about the virtue of forgiveness, and how you might develop it.

Here are some insights that might help:

2.3. The art of forgiveness, and two process models

(a) Kornfield on forgiveness

> "To err is human; to forgive, divine".
>
> Alexander Pope. From page 198 of Ratcliffe (2010).

I begin this section by reviewing some quotations from a lovely little book by Jack Kornfield[13], which I have found very helpful in my own life:

On page 22 of this book, Kornfield describes a conversation between two former prisoners of war. The first one asks the other one if he has *forgiven his captors* yet. The second one said **definitely not**. Then the first one says: "Well, then, they still have you in prison, don't they?"

This little exchange is designed to teach us that the function of forgiveness in our lives is *to liberate ourselves*; to give ourselves a degree of *peace*; or liberation from resentment and constantly carrying angry memories of long-past insults, hurts, humiliations and other forms of suffering.

When we forgive, we can finally put all this baggage down, and let it go, and breathe freely once more!

For many years, I have been teaching these two points:

1. Indulging in resentment is like taking poison, and waiting for the other person to die. But they don't die, because we are poisoning ourselves with our bitterness! And:

2. The Buddhists teach this point: Getting angry at people who offend us is like picking up a hot coal with the intention of throwing it at our transgressor; but it is us who gets our hand burned!

As Jack Kornfield writes, "It is painful to hate".

He goes on to write: "Without forgiveness we continue to perpetuate the illusion that hate can heal our pain... (But) In forgiveness we let go and find relief in our heart". (Page 23).

On page 25, he writes this: "The past is over: Forgiveness means giving up all hope of a better past"!

However, this does not mean 'forgetting the god-awful past!' We have to take the time to remember it; process it; chew it through, and finally digest it.

Kornfield acknowledges that forgiveness does not happen quickly; and it may involve "a long process of grief, outrage, sadness, loss and pain".

We should not try to suppress or ignore our pain; or to hurry up the grieving process. It takes time.

And forgiveness should not be confused with forgetting. We should recognize when we have been treated with injustice, unfairness or malicious or negligent hurtfulness. But we should also try to "understand the conditions that brought (the suffering) about". (Page 29).

"When we forgive we can also say, 'Never again will I allow these things to happen'. We may resolve to never again permit such harm to come to ourselves or another". (Kornfield, 2002, Page 29).

Forgiveness does not deny us our self-protective urges and self-defence systems. We should try to achieve the fairest, most equal relationships with others that we can create. We should not 'roll over' in the face of injustice, unfairness, or intimidation.

~~~

(b) The 'positive psychology' of forgiveness

> *"I ain't sayin' you treated me unkind. You could have done better but I don't mind. You just kinda wasted my precious time. But don't think twice, it's all right".*

> Bob Dylan, Singer/song-writer. (1963 song: *Don't think twice, it's all right).*

In this section, I want to present a nice little model which was included in a *Positive Psychology Newsletter* on the subject of *Forgiveness,* by Dr Ben Dean, from 2005. (Ben was involved in a Happiness Coaching Program in which I participated, around 2004-2005). This model could be used by anybody, including individuals who want to forgive an ex-partner against whom they have been storing painful resentment. When relationships don't work out, you do not have to continue to relate to the other person. You can forgive them, and let them go, on the basis that they are not good for you. Even if the ex-partner tries to make amends, we do not have to naively put ourselves at risk. We are free to forgive them their transgressions, and to move on!

A Process Model of Forgiveness

Developmental psychologist Robert Enright provides a process model of forgiveness that could be applied to forgiveness interventions with individuals or groups.

In an article in the *Chronicle of Higher Education* (Heller, 1998[14]), he outlines the following nine steps toward forgiveness:

1. Acknowledge your emotions. Whether you are angry, hurt, ashamed, or embarrassed (or some combination of the above), acknowledge your emotional reaction to the wrongdoing.

2. Go beyond identifying the person who hurt you and articulate the specific behaviours that upset or hurt you.

3. Make the choice to forgive.

4. Explain to yourself why you made the decision to forgive. Your reasons can be as practical as wanting to be free of the anger so that you can concentrate better at work.

5. Attempt to "walk in the shoes" of the other person. Consider that person's vulnerabilities.

6. Make a commitment to not pass along the pain you have endured — even to the person who hurt you in the first place.

7. Decide instead to offer the world mercy and goodwill. At this stage, you may wish to reconcile with the other person (but that's not necessary – and sometimes it's not wise!)

8. Reflect on how it feels to let go of a grudge. Find meaning in the suffering you experienced and overcame.

9. Discover the paradox of forgiveness: As you give the gift of forgiveness to others, you receive the gift of peace.

~~~

(c) Anne Teachworth's Exercise for couples

Ann Teachworth is a Gestalt therapist in the USA, who has developed a wonderful insight into the way we copy our parents' relationship as a map or model for our own future relationships. In her book on couple relationships, she also presents an exercise to help individuals to learn to forgive their partner after some hurt feeling has arisen about a particular negative action.

In a journal or notebook, consider the following questions:

(a). What could your partner do – what action could they take in the future – which would cause you to forgive them?

(b). Make up a story in which your partner does actually take the action you imagined in response to the previous question.

(c). Make sure you have total privacy, and then read this story (from point 2 above) aloud.

(d). In a private space, set out three chairs, as follows:

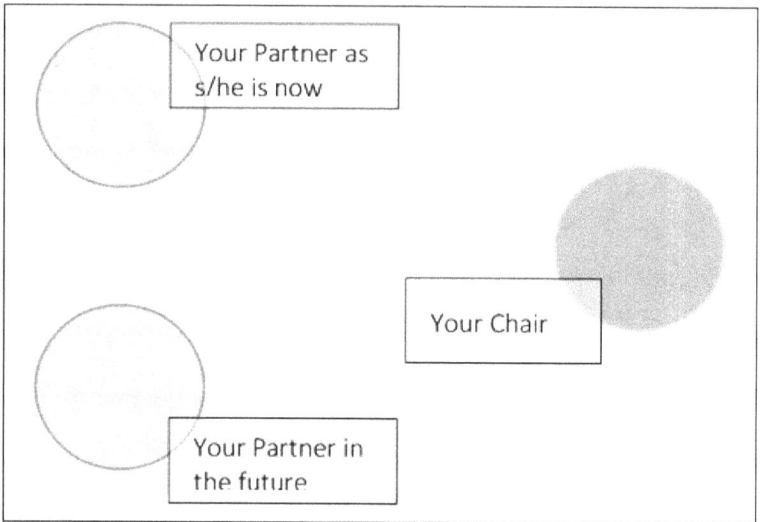

(e). Sit on your chair and look at the chair on which you imagine you can see your partner as they are now (with their hurtful behaviour – or whatever offended you – intact). Then imagine he or she gets up and moves to the "Partner in the future" chair. Look at his facial expression and body language, and see/hear him or her say the kinds of words that you want to hear (from your story in point (b) above).

(f) Now you move to that "Partner in the future" chair, and role-play your partner saying the things you want to hear, with the right kind of face and body language.

(g) Return to "Your chair", and respond to your imagined partner, on the "Partner in the future" chair, as if they had said what you wanted to hear them say.

(h) Check your bodily and mental feelings, and create the kinds of feelings that you would most likely feel, if your partner had actually said those words.

(i) Move back to your "Partner in the future" chair, and try to feel how your partner would feel if they had just said the required/desired words and then they'd heard your response.

(j) Now tell this story, of what your partner said to gain your forgiveness, and what you said in response, and what you felt and what they felt.

(k) Then, tell this same story twice more, in the past tense, as if his or her apologetic actions, and your forgiveness, had already happened, resulting in a reunion.

~~~

Summing up

Excessive or inappropriate anger mainly hurts the angry person. It is like taking poison and waiting for the other person to die. Or like picking up a rot coal with the intention of throwing at the other person, but it is our hand that gets burned!

Sometimes we can discharge our anger by being appropriately assertive. Sometimes we can reframe the transgression as being less serious than it had at first seemed. And sometimes we have to find a way to forgive the person who offended against us.

If we want to be at peace, and assertiveness and re-framing do not help; then we have to find a way to forgive those individuals and groups who have transgressed against us; harmed us; hurt us; frustrated us; or caused us pain.

Those individuals may often include our own parents, during our own childhood. Unless and until we dig up our difficult childhood memories, and learn to forgive our parents for being fallible products of their own childhood experiences, we cannot heal, and we cannot grow to be fully who we are in potential.

And then, we also have to learn to forgive ourselves for our imperfect performances in our earlier relationships; in our social roles; in politics; and in our working lives. We have to learn to forgive ourselves for the wasted time, wasted energy, and wasted potential which are an inevitable part of our slow coming to consciousness as human beings.

And we have to learn to forgive ourselves and our current and earlier partner(s) for our clumsy attempts to form relationships, which inevitably caused a good deal of pain and suffering, including jealousy, envy, anger, fear of abandonment, fear of being controlled, and much more besides.

Forgiveness may seem like an expression of weakness, but only the truly strong can forgive. Forgiveness does not mean forgetting. We may often develop stronger boundaries against future abusive or hurtful actions by forgiving somebody, and always remembering that such things could happen again in the future, but not if we resist and defend ourselves against abuse, neglect, and harm.

Forgiveness is a much more sensible option than attempting to "accept other people unconditionally". That is a recipe for strengthening their immorality, and indicating that we have weak boundaries which allow us to be abuse or exploited.

Forgiveness is the road to peace of mind. Combined with self-assertion and strong boundaries, forgiveness is an essential part of the toolkit of the emotionally intelligent individual.

And in this chapter I have outlined two processes that can be used to help you to achieve a state of forgiveness with another person: the positive psychology process model, and Anne Teachworth's model.

~~~

Chapter 3: Six ways to re-frame your anger-inducing problems

~~~

~~~

3.1: Introduction

In Chapter 12 of this book, I have argued that angry outbursts are affected by the current state of the whole body-brain-mind of the individual expressing that angry outburst. To demonstrate my point, I introduced the Holistic-SOR model, where

S = Stimulus, or what happened to the individual to induce them to become angry.

O = The total state of the person as an **Organism**. And:

R = The (appropriately or inappropriately) angry **Response**.

Within the Holistic-SOR model - (reproduced in the Figure on the next page) - in the middle column, what we are aiming to do is to construct a balance sheet (in our heads) of the *pressures* bearing down on the client (person), and the *coping resources* that they have for dealing with those pressures.

~~~

So this is a *historical-social-stress model*.

It is not a purely 'cognitive distortion' model; nor a purely 'biological/ sexual urges' model;

Nor a purely 'prizing and listening' model.

Indeed, it is the most holistic model of human functioning that has ever appeared in published form, to the best of my knowledge and belief.

The Holistic Stimulus-Organism-Response Model (H-SOR)		
Column 1	Column 2	Column 3
S = Stimulus	O = Organism	R = Response
When something significant happens, which is apprehended by the organism's (or person's) nervous system, the organism is activated or aroused (positively or negatively)	The organism responds, well or badly. The incoming stimulus may activate or interact with: (1) Innate needs and tendencies; (2) Family history and attachment style; (3) Recent personal history; (4) Emotive-cognitive schemas (as guides to action); (5) Narratives, stories, frames and other storied elements (which may be hyper-activating, hypo-activating, or affect regulating); (6) Character and temperament; (7) Need satisfaction; goals and values; (8) Diet and supplementation, medication, exercise regime, sleep and relaxation histories; (9) Ongoing environmental stressors, state of current relationship(s), and satisfaction with life stages, etc., etc.	The organism outputs a response, in the form of visible behaviour and inferable emotional reactions, like anger, anxiety, depression, embarrassment, etc.

The Holistic SOR Model of E-CENT origin

~~~

3.2: Anger triggers

A particular Stimulus, or trigger, will result in a particular Response, depending upon the total state of the Organism (person).

But what kinds of triggers typically elicit an angry response?

We explore that question in the table on the next page:

Neglect	Abandonment	Abuse
Exploitation	Oppression	Being overly-controlled
Threat (which is not excessive, and is surmountable)	Frustration	Insulting words or behaviour
Breaking of moral rules, or personal rules	Cheating or short-changing	Unfairness
Disrespect	Being criticized	Being blamed unfairly
Being interrupted in conversation	Being patronized	

Of course, not everybody who is treated unfairly, or frustrated, will respond with anger. That depends upon the state of the individual's body-brain-mind, based on all the factors listed above, when we considered the Holistic-SOR model.

~~~

3.3: There's more to life than philosophy

Sometimes working on a person's philosophy of life will help them to reduce or control their anger; but they also normally have to work on their body, via physical fitness, adequate nutrition, sufficient good-quality sleep, and various other factors.

For example:

- Eating junk foods, high in trans-fats, has been shown to cause individuals to develop anger management problems.

- By contrast, introducing young, violent prisoners to a diet high in omega-3 fats, has been found to reduce incidents of violence or aggressive conflict dramatically.

And depending on what your childhood was like, you may also have to go back and dig up some aspects of your past history; meaning your historical relationships with your mother, father, siblings, teachers, peers, and so on: and to rewrite or revise stressful or traumatic experiences that were left undigested at the time. (See Appendix D).

~~~

But philosophy of life is also important. And if you think your diet, sleep and exercise are not contributing much to your current problem of anger; and that it is not about unresolved problems from your earlier life; then it makes sense to work on how you perceive insults, frustrations, potential harm, or other hurtful behaviours by the people with whom you have to relate.

~~~

3.4: Frames and framing: Perspectives on life's difficulties

When an E-CENT counsellor sets out to work on the philosophy of life of an angry client, they normally utilize the EFR model. This is it:

E = Event = What happened, or what happens? (See the list of potential triggers above).

F = Frame or Framing = The client will have applied *a non-conscious frame of reference* to the interpretation of the event (E). And:

R = Response = A total body-brain-mind state of angry arousal. (This is an expression of the so-called 'fight response'.

So let us look more closely at the concept of 'frame' or 'framing'.

According to my English Dictionary, the word frame refers to things like picture frame; door frame; spectacle frame; building or car frame; the human (body) frame; but this is not the sense in which I am using the concept of frame in this chapter. And then we get this:

"...5. The underlying structure that supports a system or idea". Soanes (2002)[15].

This is a bit closer, because I am trying to point to the fact that, underneath any *interpretation* is a structure of concepts.

So let us take a look at the definition of 'frame' from my dictionary of psychology:

"...2. An underlying *assumption* or set of assumptions that supports an interpretation or a concept and that functions as *an interpretive frame of reference* for thinking about the concept..."

An example of interpretive frame of reference cold be this: If you are out walking in the street, and a friend of yours walks past you without saying hello, you might automatically conclude that "He must not like me anymore!" (That is just an automatic interpretation, based on a particular frame of reference).

If I had a similar experience with a friend of mind tomorrow, I might automatically interpret their lack of communication with me to the idea that "he is obviously very preoccupied".

And other individuals might come up with various other interpretations, based on their habitual frames of reference for such an experience.

So, we could now say that "...a frame is a knowledge structure of an everyday aspect of the world..." (Colman, 2002)[16].

So, a frame, in our present context, is *an interpretive frame of reference, or the knowledge structure that allows us to know how to interpret a particular signal* coming into our senses, of sight, sound, touch, etc. (And our interpretative frames may be helpful and insightful, or unhelpful and misleading).

For example, when somebody insults you, with a particular form of words, you already have a 'frame of reference' stored in the non-conscious part of your brain-mind, which dictates *how you will see/hear that insult*, and *how you will feel* about that insult, and what you will feel like *doing* about that insult. To change your *philosophy of life* about anger-inducing signals means to change your 'frames of reference' about anger-inducing signals. The Six Windows Model of E-CENT offers six new 'frames of reference' which allow you to escape from your habit-based tendency to over-react to insults, frustrations, insults and to people who 'break the rules'.

~~~

3.5: Introducing the Six Windows Model

I originally created a *Four Windows model*, back in 2007-9, as I moved away from the Extreme Stoicism of Rational Therapy (REBT). Later I added a fifth window, and then Renata added the sixth window.

The Six Windows Model of E-CENT counselling is a way of helping clients to rethink and re-frame their noxious problems, without engaging in confrontation and heated arguments.

It consists of *an experiment*, in which the angry client is *asked* to imagine how their problem would look when viewed through six different window frames – each of which provides a slightly different 'frame of reference' for *interpreting* the problem.

Here's how it works:

Let us take the increasingly common problem of 'road rage', in which a frustrated driver, stuck behind a slow-moving vehicle, becomes more and more angry, until they explode and take risky action to overtake the slower driver.

Imagine you are that frustrated driver, and you've been stuck behind a slow-moving vehicle – like a farm tractor – for several miles, and you are going to be late for an important meeting because of this delay.

Now look through each of the following six 'windows' in turn, (as if looking at that serious problem of frustration and delay), and ask yourself the questions suggested:

~~~

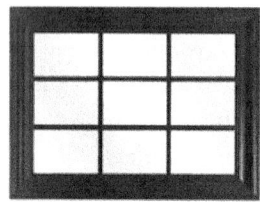

Window No.1: This window has the following (realistic) assumption written around the frame: "Life is **difficult** *for all human beings*, at least some of the time, and often much of the time".

Imagine you believe that assumption (or frame) and that you are looking out through this window at your problem of being stuck behind a slow-moving tractor, and ask yourself the following questions:

1. "If life is difficult for all humans at least some of the time, and I am a human, isn't it obvious that life is going to be difficult for me at least some of the time?" (Your answer has to be 'yes'!)

So, following on from that point,

2. "Why must it not be difficult for me right now (being stuck behind this slow-moving tractor, and being obliged to be late for my important meeting)?"

It is obvious that it has to be difficult for you right now. If you are feeling angry at the tractor driver, then you are applying an insupportable 'frame of reference' to inform your interpretation.

Perhaps you have been wired up by your own socialized experience to believe: "there should never be any traffic delays when I am in a hurry!" But that is clearly unrealistic, unreasonable and somewhat mad; since it is (almost by definition) on those occasions when you badly need to **not** be delayed that you get angry about being delayed, because you hardly notice those delays when you are not in such a hurry. So, ask yourself:

3. "Is there any realistic reason to believe that there should not be any traffic jams when I am in a hurry?" (The answer is obviously 'no'!)

And isn't it also the case that you are angry at the slow driver in front because you are *projecting the blame* onto him (or her) for your late arrival at the impending meeting, when, in point of fact, *you are the one who is responsible* because you did not plan for any delays when you set out to get to this important meeting.

Two changes to your *philosophy* and *practical management* of your life will eliminate your angry frustrations and your tendency to road rage:

1. Try teaching yourself this truth, over and over again, day after day, week after week, and month after month:

> "Since I am a human, it follows that I will experience difficulties! Because life is difficult for all human beings at least some of the time, and often much of the time".

So stop railing against the inevitable. It serves no useful function, and harms you in many ways.

2. Also, notice those situations in which you get angry and take responsibility for your anger, *instead of **blaming** others*. In this present illustration, you need to teach yourself *to always **pad** your journey time* to allow for what seems to inevitably happen from time to time: inevitable (but unpredictable) delays. It is inevitable that, from time to time you will be delayed; and so you should *always* pad your journey time when travelling to important meetings, even if that means that, more often than not, you arrive *too early*. (You can always teach yourself to make good use of the time you have in hand when you arrive early!)

~~~

Window No.2: The realistic assumption written around this frame is as follows:

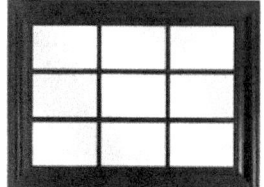

"Life is **significantly less difficult,** provided I avoid picking and choosing unrealistic outcomes; or if I pick and choose *more sensibly* or *reasonably.*"

The *extreme Stoics* used to try to teach their followers to give up *all forms of picking and choosing.* But this is unrealistic and unachievable for almost all humans. However, what we can do is to give up *extreme forms* of picking and choosing: like insisting that the roads should always be clear when we are in a hurry.

Ask yourself the following three questions, when you imagine yourself stuck behind that slow moving tractor, on the way to your very important meeting:

1. "Is it realistic to expect that this tractor should not have turned up here this morning, just because I am in a hurry?"

(The answer is obviously 'no'!)

2. "Is it sensible for me to think that, if I allow myself to become very angry, and red in the face, and start shouting inaudibly in the soundproofed interior of my car, that the tractor driver will realize that s/he has to pull over and get out of my way?"

(Of course not!)

3. "And is it realistic to assume that, if I tailgate the tractor, and blow my car horn repeatedly, that the tractor driver *will* find a way to pull over and let me through?"

(Probably not! So you should put this down to experience, accept responsibility for being late; and pad my journey time in future, especially when you are driving to a very important meeting!)

You should also teach yourself the following frame of reference, by reviewing it over and over and over again, for 30, 60 or 90 days:

"Life is **significantly less difficult,** provided I avoid picking and choosing unrealistic outcomes; or if I pick and choose *more sensibly* or *reasonably.*"

~~~

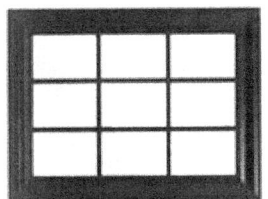

Window No.3: This window has the following realistic assumption written around the frame: "Life is **both** difficult **and** non-difficult".

Imagine you believe this assumption, and you are looking out through this window at the tractor blocking your way. Then, ask yourself these questions:

1. "Is my anger entirely to do with this tractor driver blocking my way forward? Or is it partly due to the fact that I have tunnel vision on this problem? If I split my attention between this delay in my journey, and some things for which I could be grateful, would I be likely to feel less angry?"

If you are very angry about being stuck behind this tractor when you are in a hurry to get to an important meeting, might it not be because you are *exclusively* focusing on the difficulties, and overlooking those bits which are *not* difficult (for which you could be grateful)?

What could you be grateful for?

1. You could appreciate the insight that you have to *normally* pad your journey times to allow for such *occasionally* unavoidable traffic jams. (If you learn this lesson well, there is no need to ever find yourself in this kind of traffic delay in the future; barring real emergencies!)

2. You should be grateful that you are stuck in a traffic *jam*, and not in a traffic *pile-up*, in which you have been injured.

3. You may have a mobile phone (cell phone) in your car, so you be grateful that you can phone ahead and make the best excuse you can for your expected degree of lateness!

4. This could be the moment when you realize that you should not spoil the peace and calm of *the present moment* for any assumed or real benefit in the future! The present moment is *all the time we have*, and we have to learn to enjoy it, sooner or later.

You could benefit a lot from teaching yourself this principle, value or philosophical stance:

"Life is **both** difficult **and** non-difficult".

Review that slogan or belief over and over again, day after day, week after week, and month after month, until you could recite it in your sleep!

So do not waste your time and energy focusing exclusively on the difficult bits. Remember to include the non-difficult bits. And enjoy the moment!

~~~

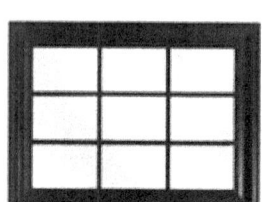

Window No.4: This frame has the following realistic slogan or assumption written around it:

"Life could always be *very much more difficult* than it currently is for me".

Ask yourself these questions:

1. "Am I making the mistake of thinking that it's going to be 100% bad to be late for this meeting?" (It may be a high percentage, but probably not 100%)

2. "If I think it's 100% bad to be late for this meeting, what percentage would I apply to the possibility that my engine could overheat, and I might not get to my destination until tomorrow, instead of early today?" (There is nothing higher than 100% - even though it is now commonplace for people to claim that they give 110% to their jobs!)

3. "If I think it's 100% bad to be late for this meeting, what percentage would I apply to the possibility that I could cause myself a heart attack, or a bleeding ulcer, by stewing in my own angry juices?" And:

4. "What if a crocodile was eating my rear end off, in addition to my being stuck behind this tractor, what percentage would that be?"

You could benefit from teaching yourself the following principle, by reading it a few times each day, for 30, 60, or 90 days, to get it into your long-term memory:

"Life could always be *very much more difficult* than it currently is for me".

~~~

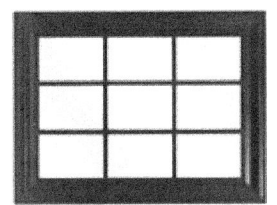

Window No.5: The reasonable assumption which is written around this frame is as follows:

"In life, there are certain things I can control, and certain things that are beyond my control".

Imagine you believe this slogan, and that you are looking our through this window at the traffic delay ahead. Ask yourself:

1. "Am I currently upset because I am **trying** to control something that is **beyond** my control?" (Certainly, it does not seem to be realistic to try to shunt this tractor out of your way. You have tried beeping your car horn; and tailgating the offending vehicle, without any success).

2. "If I give up trying to control what is clearly beyond my control, how much happier will I feel?" (In my experience, you would feel a lot happier the moment you give up trying to *not be* behind the vehicle that you are *actually* behind!)

3. "Is there anything I *could* control, in this situation, which would improve the problem of being late for an important meeting?" (Could you phone ahead and let somebody know you will be late? Could you arrange something to fill the time that you will not be there, to avoid somebody having to pointlessly wait around for you? Or, should you – when the traffic comes to a total halt - write a file note in your diary about how you will always pad your journey time in future, especial when you are travelling to an important meeting, even if you think you know – based on past experiences – how long the journey 'should take'!)

And now, make a commitment to learn the following philosophical stance:

"In life, there are certain things I can control, and certain things that are beyond my control".

Review this statement over and over again, for the next month, or two or three, until you get it reliably into your long-term memory.

~~~

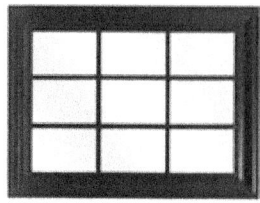 **Window No.6:** The realistic slogan or assumption written around this window is as follows:

"If life is a school in which we can learn from experience, what positive lesson could I learn from my current negative situation?"

Imagine you believe this slogan, and that you are looking out through this window at the tractor moving slowly ahead of you.

Now ask yourself:

1. "What *positive lesson* could I possibly learn from this *negative* experience?" (You could learn to always pad your journey time, especially on important journeys. You could learn that you have to accept the things you cannot change. You could learn that you have a tendency to see every frustration as 100% bad, when they are often very much less than that!)

2. "What does this situation teach me about the source or nature of my anger management problem? (It could teach you that *you do not plan ahead*; that you do not *plan for emergencies*; that you are *too complacent* about the speed of your car and the ease of access of the network of roads. That you are *too easily upset* by relatively minor problems and frustrations! Being late for an important meeting is relatively minor, compared with the problems that eighty percent of the population of planet Earth have to face on a daily basis – like grinding poverty; sickness and disease; military dictatorship; lack of personal power, and lack of political influence; and so on.

~~~

Reflection:

Did this process, of viewing a current problem from six different 'directions' or perspectives; or through six different 'lenses', or 'frames'; change how it looks and feels to you? (Normally it will!)

Did your anger level fall? (Normally it will!)

Did you learn any valuable lessons? (Normally you will!)

~~~

Study tips

If you read this chapter just once, then what you learn will be limited, and it will also quickly drain from your memory banks. If you value this Six Windows approach, then you owe it to yourself to learn it properly. That can be done by reading this chapter at least three times:

❒ First reading

❒ Second reading

❒ Third reading

Make notes in a journal or notebook of the key points that you are learning, as you go along.

When you run into an anger-inducing problem in your life, sit down with your notebook or journal, and write it up:

> **E = Event** = What happened?
>
> **F = Framing**. This is non-conscious, so you are unlikely to know what it is, though you may sometimes be able to make inferences (or informed guesses) about what it could have been. (For example: "Life is denying me what I want and need! This is totally bad! Somebody has to 'pay' for this" [in the sense of being punished!])
>
> **R = Response** = Anger = On a scale of 1-10, just how angry were you?

Then: Apply the Six Windows Model to that problem, looking through each of the six windows in turn, and writing down the questions – shown above (in each Window section) – and answering them for yourself.

In this way, you will slowly change your philosophy of life, becoming much more reasonable when faced by frustrations, difficulties, insults, abusive words or treatment, threats, and so on.

However, do bear in mind that there will be occasions when there are things you can control about the situation, and on those occasions it is important to change the things you can. Sometimes, this requires you to act assertively with another person. (See Appendix C).

~~~

Get your anger under reasonable control

Part 2: More detailed introduction and definitions

Part 2 consists of Chapters 4 and 5, which cover the process of defining anger; and introducing a range of psychological models of anger.

This builds up to the presentation of our emotive-cognitive model, as follows:

The E-CENT* model shows why it is not enough to ask an angry person "What are you *telling yourself* about (X) in order to *make yourself* angry?" It is not enough to look at their thinking, or their philosophy of life. Most often they will not know what they thought-felt-perceived, immediately before becoming angry. They will not know the 'frames' they are viewing the problem through, because those frames are non-conscious and automatic.

And, by the same token, it is not *enough* - not sufficient - to ask a client what their negative automatic thoughts happen to be, because their thoughts do *not* cause their emotions.

This is so because – in addition to their philosophy of life - the person's anger level is partly driven by their emotional sensitivity (which is genetically determined); partly by the culture and sub-culture(s) from which they come (because of social learning); and partly from their physiological state resulting from their use, or lack of use, of physical exercise, healthy diet, stimulants, medicines, and adequate amounts of good quality sleep; and much more besides.

~~~

*E-CENT = Emotive-Cognitive Embodied Narrative Therapy.

~~~

Get your anger under reasonable control

Chapter 4: Defining anger

Introduction

In this chapter, I will begin to define anger more clearly and precisely; deal with its innate nature; and its constructive and destructive aspects. And then I will present an exploration of the emotive-cognitive (E-CENT) theory of anger.

~~~

Beginning to define anger

> "Acute, explosive anger is potentially harmful because it generates destructive behaviours and alienates other people. Less intense but more sustained anger is also self-defeating because it drains our energy, impairs our relationships, makes us unhappy and can adversely affect our health". Dr Sarah Edelman (2006)[17].

~~~

According to my English dictionary, 'anger' means: "A strong feeling of extreme displeasure".[18]

And Fisher (2005) says that "Anger is a feeling – nothing more and nothing less. It is no more inherently 'good' or 'bad' than any other feeling"[19]. It is what we do with our anger that makes for good or bad outcomes, and moral or immoral action.

Darwin saw anger as related to dislike and/or hatred of another:

"If we have suffered or expect to suffer some wilful injury from a (wo)man, or if s/he is in any way offensive to us, we dislike him (or her); and dislike easily rises into hatred. Such feelings, if experienced in a moderate degree, are not clearly expressed by any movement of the body or features, excepting perhaps by a certain gravity of behaviour, or by some ill-temper. Few individuals, however, can long reflect about a hated person, without feeling and exhibiting signs of indignation or rage"[20].

Anger is natural and innate

Anger has been widely agreed to be universal, natural and innate, since Darwin's book was published in 1898; but it is also culturally shaped[21]. It is most often, in its healthy form, an expression of frustration at goal blockage, seen in infants from the early months of life[22]. Infants can identify anger from about the age of ten weeks old; and they become capable of expressing anger in the first year of life, potentially to the detriment of their relationships with parents[23].

Anger is also, as implied by Darwin above, often seen as a strong negative emotion against someone; a response to insult, injury, mistreatment, opposition, frustration, or other threats to one's goals or one's self esteem.

Anger can be expressed openly as *verbal* or *physical* aggression; rage; or hostility; or in a *passive* form, such as sulking, or trying indirectly to hurt the person or thing that is perceived as the attacker – often referred to as a passive-aggressive response[24]. But it can also be expressed *appropriately*, meaning assertively, constructively, or in spontaneous self-defence when physically attacked.

Some theorists mistakenly believe anger is *always* wrong: an expression of the negative aspects of a human ego. However, since anger can be found throughout the animal kingdom, it seems not to be solely about ego so much as a perceived threat to surviving or thriving. (Darwin, 1898; and Lorenz, 1966). Of course, in the case of humans, the question of ego does arise: we want to look good, in our own eyes, and the eyes of others. Therefore, anybody who threatens our self-concept, or ego image, is perceived as threatening our interests. Any threat to what a person considers to be their 'personal domain' is likely to produce some degree of hostile response.

Anger can be constructive or destructive

Some theorists correctly consider that anger can be either constructive or destructive[25]; and this is especially so in the case of counselling and therapy systems, and assertiveness training. For example, behaviour modification therapy teaches self-assertion to its clients, so they can use an appropriate amount of their innate aggression to defend their personal space, while, at the same time, respecting the personal space of those individuals with whom they communicate, including those with whom they assertively communicate. Gestalt therapists also consider that innate aggression is important, for example in 'chewing through' our interpersonal experiences.

Of course, when people use anger and aggression *inappropriately*, they hurt others, or offend them, and cause a backlash that often works to the detriment of the angry individual.

On the other hand, the angry person may not be punished by the other for their aggressive words or deeds, but a little while later the angry person calms down, and now feels guilty, ashamed and stupid because of the things they said or did in the heat of rageful reaction.

Furthermore, immediately after a person makes him/herself angry at, and communicates that anger to, another person, the angry person may flip into anxiety or fear, in anticipation of a backlash from the victim of their angry outburst.

Apart from inducing guilt, shame and fear, inappropriate anger can result in broken relationships, lost jobs, lost friends, arrest for actual bodily harm, legal prosecution, fines, imprisonment, community service, stomach ulcers (as we stew in our own angry juices), damage to our heart and arteries, poor relations with our neighbours, loss of peace of mind (as our mind spins in hot rage and dreams of revenge), loss of happiness, loss of social status (as we show up more and more like a petulant child, or a bully!), loss of face, loss of self-respect and respect from others.

~~~

Exploring the E-CENT theory of anger

The E-CENT theory of anger says that anger is one of our basic emotions. It's innate. It was selected by nature for its survival value. We would not survive for long without an innate sense of *angering* in response to abuse or neglect. We also would not survive for long if we did not quickly learn how to *moderate* our anger as young children.

My anger (like yours) is a two-edged sword. It can help to protect me, and it can attract hostile reactions from others.

My **basic** emotion of anger (like yours) is elaborated into a *higher cognitive emotion* through modelling by my mother and father and significant others in the first few years of my life. My ability to become *emotionally intelligent* in relation to my innate anger urges depends on the emotional intelligence of my parents. My first angry outbursts are with them. How successfully I and they handle those angry episodes will shape how I manage my anger in the school playground. And my socialized anger management strategies continue to evolve through my successful and my unsuccessful experiences of engaging in conflict with others: siblings, school peers, and so on.

I may become an *exploder*, who erupts in the faces of others.

I may become an *imploder*, who keeps his anger inside.

Or I may hide my anger from myself (repress it) and then project it into my environment where it may frighten me.

So anger is a socialized emotion, and if you grew up with angry people, you are likely to be prone to angering yourself when provoked; or you might feel fearful of your own anger, or the anger of others.

~~~

Healthy anger is present-time defence of your legitimate rights in the face of inappropriate behaviour by another person. Healthy or *reasonable* anger is the fuel that drives our *assertive* behaviours. It pushes us to engage in *constructive conflict*, when that is **necessary**!

To ask for what you want, which is legitimately yours to request, requires a certain level of 'fire in your belly'. If you lack that fire (that *reasonable* level of anger), then you will tend to 'wimp-out'; to act passively and let other people control you, or intimidate you, or deny you your reasonable share of the social stage. One of the problems that we encounter in therapy is this: Some parents, anxious to socialize their children to be 'nice' and 'civilized', go too far in 'switching off their fierceness' – instead of teaching them to manage their fierceness appropriately. And one of the things we do for passive clients is to help them to switch on their 'fierceness switch' – but to only use their fierceness *assertively*, up to the boundary of their personal space – and never to invade the personal space of another – or to use their fierceness *aggressively*!

Unhealthy or *unreasonable* anger is an over-reaction to a frustrating or insulting stimulus from another person or external force. Unhealthy or unreasonable anger leads to *aggressive* actions and destructive conflict. It is an *excessive* use of fierceness, and an under-use of communication and negotiation strategies.

We teach the following eight insights to our anger management clients:

1. You were born with *an **innate capacity** to develop angry*, anxious and depressed responses to your social environment - in response to frustrations, threats and losses.

2. You then encountered your mother, who already had a 'style of relating', based on her attachment experience of relating to her own mother and father (when she was a child). She would inevitably have shaped your emotional expression by:

> (a) Modelling an approach to relationship and emotions; and:

> (b) Rewarding and penalizing you for your daily emotion expressions, including your angry outbursts in the first couple of years of your life.

3. Your father's approach to relationship, including emotion expression, especially his way of expressing (or suppressing) anger, would have been the next major influence on the development of your emotion expression, including your way of being angry - implosive or explosive; direct or indirect; passive or aggressive; appropriate or inappropriate.

4. If both of your parents had a secure attachment to their own parents, they would have had a warm but assertive approach to relating to you. From them you would have learned to be secure in your relationship with them, and, by extension, in virtually all subsequent people-encounters. You would have learned to express healthy or appropriate anger in an *assertive* way - to ask for what you want, and to say no to what you do not want. And to strive to be treated with respect as an equal human being. You would not have any significant problems with anger.

5. However, if one or both of your parents had an insecure attachment to their own parents, they would have had an insecure attachment to you, and been either explosively or implosively angry with you when you frustrated them or broke their *personal* rules, or their *culturally shaped moral rules*. From them, you would have learned to engage in unhealthy or inappropriate anger expression of an explosive or implosive type, or a mixture of the two, varying from situation to situation. (Or you might have learned to be *passive* in those situations in which you felt frightened or fearful of reprisals, but *aggressive* in those situations where you felt no constraint of fearfulness!)

6. If you want to change your relationship style today, you need to experience a secure relationship with another person - possibly a romantic partner; a very good friend; or a good therapist who understands how to build a secure relationship with you. You need to learn the difference between *appropriate* and *inappropriate* anger. And you also could benefit from learning that **explosive** anger - (like shouting and using aggressive body language) - costs you, in terms of damage to relationships and careers, for examples; and that *implosive anger* – (like sulking and stewing in your own angry juices, or withdrawing aggressively) - damages your ongoing happiness, your relationships at home and at work, and ultimately your physical and mental health.

7. You can improve your relationship and attachment style by studying and applying new ideas from emotional literacy and self-assertion. And I (and/or other counsellors) can teach those ideas and skills to you. (See Appendices 'B' and 'C' below).

8. But you are also a body-mind, and so your approach to managing your diet, physical exercise, sleep pattern, self-talk (or inner dialogue), and relaxation/ meditation, are also important. And it is easier to develop a secure attachment style if your romantic partner is already secure.

~~~

When an E-CENT counsellor works with an angry client, they may work on deep, emotional and attachment issues from early childhood; or on present-time assertiveness skills; or advice on important dietary changes; or recommendations regarding regular physical exercise, or improvements to sleep patterns; or teaching the client how to reframe their anger-inducing experiences; or changing some elements of their philosophy of life (as they show up in their inner dialogues about anger-inducing situations) – and even to change some aspect of their social or physical environment with which they have been putting up or tolerating unnecessarily!

~~~

Chapter 5: Psychological models of emotion

"We respond physically to the (anger inducing) stimulus, exhibiting the bodily changes which accompany the tension that is generated when we are faced with a threat. Then we develop angry thoughts and feelings, which influence how we behave". Hartley (2002)[26].

~~~

Since anger is a human (and wider animal) emotion, we must firstly look to psychology for our understanding of emotions, including anger. Unfortunately, cognitive psychology has largely ignored emotion, while focusing its attention on the *thinking processes* of the human mind (as if thinking and feeling could be separated out from each other, which they can not!) Because of this error of judgement, made by early psychologists, the main field of cognitive psychology has focused upon: attention, perception, memory, language and thinking. (A tiny element of consideration of emotion was tacked on late in the day).

Modern science in general reflects this bias towards thinking, as opposed to emoting. For example, in Anthony Smith's 1984 book on the mind[27], there is not a single reference to emotion, affect, feelings, anger, anxiety, etc., in the index or the contents page.

By 2000, small elements of discussion of emotion were beginning to find their way into cognitive psychology texts. For example, Eysenck and Keane's book[28] contains a chapter (number 19) on 'Cognition and Emotion'. This was a radical break with the past.

Cognitive models of emotion

Eysenck and Keane present evidence which suggests that individuals with problems with anxiety tend to have:

(1) an **attentional bias** – which means they focus their attention on, and look for, threats and dangers in their environment; and:

(2) an **interpretive bias** – which causes them to exaggerate the intensity of the threats or dangers that they find.

Similar conclusions could be drawn about people who suffer with strong or uncontrollable feelings of anger.

It should be noted here that those attentional and interpretive biases are underpinned by emotions, feeling or affects, stored in bodily states, including neurological circuits. (Le Doux, 1996; Damasio, 1994; Ekman, 1993; Siegel, 2015; Schore, 2003; and Hill, 2015).

However, it is probably not just an attentional bias and an interpretive bias that keeps people angry. Many people seem to be addicted to anger because it "feels good". (This is "self-righteousness" in action. And it is also an example of "poor affect regulation" ability, based on what went on in the early relationship between the child and its mother, and later its father.) Also, since humans are *creatures of habit*, those individuals who learn angry *habits* in their family of origin will tend to carry those habits into their adult lives, unless and until they run into *a good reason* to work hard at changing those habits!

In broader undergraduate psychology courses, emotion gets more consideration than in the world of cognitive psychology. For example, in Kagan and Segal's introduction to psychology for undergraduate students[29], there are chapters on emotions and drives; motives; personality; stress; abnormal psychology; and methods of therapy and treatment; much of which has been added, or expanded, since the previous edition.

Three basic theories of emotion

In the more general psychology texts, we find a range of theories of emotion. These include:

(a) **Somatic theories**, such as those developed by James and Lange[30], which see the body as the primary source of emotion;

(b) **Neurobiological theories**, which see the brain as the seat of emotion; and:

(c) **Cognitive theories**, which see appraisal or evaluation (of a stimulus) as the cause of emotion.

The somatic theories, which began with William James, assume that emotions (including anger) are bodily responses to external events. Although this view has been in long-term decline, it has gained renewed credence due to supportive neurobiological studies by Joseph Le Doux[31] and Antonio Damasio[32].

By contrast, Cannon and Bard argued that the individual first generates a mental emotion, which then produces bodily behaviour.[33]

The neurobiological theories focus on emotion as pleasing or displeasing experiences located in the 'limbic system' (or emotion centres) of the brain, but with links to the body.

Cognitive theories, like those of Richard Lazarus[34], assume that an emotion only becomes possible after an external event is appraised and evaluated, and judged to be good ('for me') or bad ('for me'). In Rational Emotive Behaviour Therapy, the sequence is:

(a) External event > (b) Internal belief system > (c.1) Emotional response > (c.2) Behavioural response. Or, in the simple A>B>C model:

A (or **activating** event) = something bad happens to a person.

B (or **belief** system) = the person appraises and evaluates the event.

C (or emotional/behaviour **consequence**) = the person feels an emotional consequence which is given by the perceived seriousness of 'A' multiplied by the intensity of 'B'.

However, I have written an extensive critique of this ABC model in Byrne (2017)[35]; and I've created a more advanced model of the human body-brain-mind-environment complexity.

The new, integrative, E-CENT model

In Emotive-Cognitive Embodied Narrative Therapy (E-CENT), we have moved beyond this simple A>B>C model, and integrated all three of the somatic, neurobiological and cognitive theories above – plus attachment theory - into a new, more complex model, which seems to us to fit the facts better than any preceding model. The E-CENT perspective is much more in line with the following statement by Dr Robert Winston:

"According to Joseph LeDoux, a prominent researcher into human emotions – and author of *The Emotional Brain* and *Synaptic Self* – the emotional process is a body-brain interaction, the bulk of which remains buried below conscious view. The conscious 'felt' element is merely the tip of the iceberg…" (Page 138)[36].

In a later section, below, we shall set out how to understand, describe and control anger using this new, E-CENT model.

The E-CENT model shows why it is not enough to ask an angry person "What are you telling yourself about (X) in order to make yourself angry?" This is so because the person's anger level is partly driven by their emotional sensitivity (which is genetically determined); partly by the culture and sub-culture(s) from which they come (because of social learning); and partly from their physiological state resulting from their use, or lack of use, of physical exercise, healthy diet, stimulants, medicines, and adequate amounts of good quality sleep; and much more besides.

Thus E-CENT takes into account the various potential sources of anger of the individual, while REBT mainly focuses on their self-talk.

See also the section on E-CENT below, for the complex A>B>C presentation.

~~~

Part 3: Schools of thought on the subject of anger

Part 3 of this book contains eight chapters, each of which reviews the approach to anger adopted and developed by various schools of thought, including:

Chapter 6: Freud, Lorenz and Bandura on Aggression

Chapter 7: Attachment Relationships, Anger and Emotional Self-Management

Chapter 8: The Neurobiological Perspective

Chapter 9: The Stoic Perspective on Anger

Chapter 10: The Buddhist Perspective on Anger

Chapter 11. The General Cbt Position on Anger

Chapter 12: The E-Cent Theory of Anger; And:

Chapter 13: The 'Human Givens' Approach To Anger.

~~~

Get your anger under reasonable control

Chapter 6: Freud, Lorenz and Bandura on aggression

> *"…far from being the diabolical, destructive principle that classical psychoanalysis made it out to be, (aggression) is really an essential part of the life-preserving organization of instincts…"* (Lorenz, 1966/2002, page 44)[37].

~~~

Let us now look beyond the psychology of emotion, to psycho-biology, ethology and social psychology of aggression.

Beginning with Freud's theory

Sigmund Freud, who had studied much anthropology and mythology, (but also neurology), put forward the idea that human beings are driven by two main drives – one towards life and one towards death[38]. He wanted to show how his theory linked solidly to biology, at a time when biology seemed like an impressive science not just of human life, but all life. He therefore posited two sets of instincts which he believed to exist in all forms of living matter from the beginning of time – the instincts that gave rise to the emergence and growth of life forms, which he thought were broadly 'sexual' (in a quite 'non-sexual' kind of way!) – and the instincts that moved living forms towards their death[39].

He also saw the life urges as good and the death urges as bad, and for him: "Life would consist in the manifestations of the conflict or interaction between the two classes of instincts (towards life and towards death); (and) death would mean for the individual *the victory of the destructive instincts*, but reproduction would mean for him the victory of Eros (or the life instincts)". (Freud, 1993, page 157).

Just to be totally clear, let us quote him saying that the "death instincts" would "manifest themselves as destructive or aggressive impulses". (ibid, page 157).

On this account, aggression is wholly destructive, negative and life denying. However, in the E-CENT perspective, aggression (of reasonable and proportional levels) may often prove to be positive, constructive, and life enhancing.

(According to Mosby's Medical Dictionary, 'constructive aggression' is defined like this: "...an act of self-assertiveness in response to a threatening action for purposes of self-protection and preservation".[40] And it is not just because I use the prefix 'constructive' that 'aggression' comes out with a positive definition. Aggression has both a positive and a negative aspect, as indicated by the same source.[41])

Thus the E-CENT view seems to have more in common with Konrad Lorenz than with Sigmund Freud.

(We do, however, [echoing Freud], have a theory of a split in the innate character of human beings – between what the Cherokee people called the Good and Bad Wolf; and which European cultures classify as virtue and vice – but we see the defining characteristic of the Bad Wolf as harming others *unnecessarily*, and pursuing self-interest at the expense of the vital interests of others. We would see a woman hitting a man over the head with a golf club, because he was trying to rape her, as a manifestation of her Good Wolf; while if she hit him, in the same way, with the same golf club, because the engagement ring he offered her was too small, then we would see that as a manifestation of her Bad Wolf. Clearly, it is not the fact that she used aggression that makes it a Bad act, but the general context of her action. Thus aggression can be positive or negative, depending on the context).

Konrad Lorenz on aggressive instincts as evolutionarily adaptive

One of the major theorists who produced scientific evidence which overturned some of Freud's theories, was Konrad Lorenz and we agree with some of his key findings. But we also have reservations about Lorenz, as well as agreeing with some of his observations.

Konrad Lorenz was a famous scientist, and a 1973 Nobel Prize winning ethologist (which is a kind of zoologist, who studied animal behaviour). His work was based on highly detailed observations of animals – for examples: Graylag geese, jackdaws, and (in the opening of his book *On Aggression*,[42]) coral fish, which he studied in a laboratory, and in the Florida Keys.

In the first three chapters of his book on aggression, Lorenz identified three functions of aggressive behaviour in animals which promoted preservation of the species: "Namely:

(a) "balanced distribution of animals of the same species over the available environment", by driving each other away,

(b) "selection of the strongest by rival fights", which ensures that the strongest males get the best chance to mate and reproduce, "and:

(c) defence of the young" by strong, dominant animals. (Page 40).

However, he did not consider that these were the only important functions. In fact, he believed that a great part was played by aggression, for example, in motivation. And that it may fuel useful behaviour patterns that do not look anything like aggressive behaviours. For example, he considers that there is a considerable amount of aggression in the most intimate relationships between living creatures.

One important point that he makes is that it is easier to study aggression *between* animals, including humans, than it is to study, understand and expound on the role of aggression in "the interaction of drives *within* the organism". (Page 40).

So we can see that Lorenz emphasizes *the innate aggression of humans* by inferential extrapolation from animal studies. This seems intuitively right.

Bandura on the social learning of aggressive behaviours

In a famous study by Albert Bandura, in 1961, he and his associates looked at whether or not young children would model their behaviour on others if they saw them bashing an inflated doll. (This research became known as the 'Bobo doll experiments')[43].

Bandura's aim was to demonstrate that children witnessing aggressive behaviour by adults – an "aggressive model" (meaning a role model) - would copy that behaviour if they were given a chance to do so[44].

The results of this research were as follows: "The children who saw the aggressive model made more aggressive acts than the children who saw the non-aggressive model". (Banyard and Grayson, page 249).

Banyard and Grayson also helpfully look at what this research has to say, if anything, about the nature-nurture debate (in relation to the question of whether aggression is innate or socially learned).

This is what they conclude: "First, is aggression innate? Like all examples of the nature-nurture debate, it is very hard to get clear evidence one way or the other. This study (by Bandura et al, 1961) shows that aggressive behaviour can be learnt, but it does not offer any evidence on the question of whether some features of aggression are also innate". (Page 250).

In the section on the E-CENT perspective on anger, below, I will integrate Lorenz and Bandura, and show how they fit into the basic E-CENT model of mother/baby interactions.

~~~

> *"Once your anger is triggered, unless something happens to defuse the situation and calm you down, your angry feelings escalate as you become more aroused and move towards boiling or crisis point. This the stage at which your anger might increase until it erupts in a violent outburst".* Hartley (2002)[45].

~~~

Konrad Lorenz's book 'On Aggression' is a highly technical consideration of the evolutionary function of aggression, based on extensive animal studies – his own and those of other researchers. Some of his ideas are highly convincing, and some are questionable.

Two of his central conclusions are:

(1) Aggression serves the three functions mentioned above;

(2) Aggression is an intra-species phenomenon – i.e. it occurs within a species, and not between species. (He does not count predatory behaviour as aggression, in that hunting animals do not become 'angry' towards their prey, merely hungry; and

(3) In highly social species, like most mammals, especially primates, including humans, the aggressive intra-specific aggressive urges would prevent the continuance of social life if we did not have an innate 'inhibitor' of aggression.

I agree that aggression seems to be both a useful and a destructive element of animal nature. I agree that it is more destructive in humans than in most other animals. However, I do not agree that all animal aggression is intra-specific (or within the same species). For example, I have seen wolves kill a wild dog who threatened to come close to the carcass they were eating. They were not preying on the wild dog; they were *very angry* with it for competing with them for food!

Lorenz's (1966/2002) argument includes the idea that most animals will aggress against members of their own species, but that they will stop when the attacked individual yields or submits by showing a vulnerable body part (Pages 101, 133, 142-143). He says this no longer happens with humans because our cultural development has outstripped our innate nature, and that our innate 'inhibitor' of aggression has been overridden by the development of weapons which allow us to kill at a distance: (Pages 151, 212, and 233 onwards). In this way he can say that 'good men' engage in acts of bombing and shooting each other because they are not close enough to their victims to see them showing a vulnerable body part – yielding or submitting.

This is completely false, and has been shown to be so by the Stamford University Prison Experiment conducted by Zimbardo and his colleagues in 1972[46]. In this experiment, a group of respectable, middle class American students (who were on summer vacation) was split into two smaller groups, with one appointed as prison guards, and the other arrested and taken to a simulated prison as prisoners. The guards were given permission to behave as badly as they liked (by Zimbardo) and the experiment had to be ended after six days because the mental and physical cruelty inflicted upon the 'prisoners' (at close quarters) had become clearly unethical and immoral. The prisoners' 'vulnerable body parts' were within sight of the guards. The prisoners pleaded for mercy. The guards did not have any 'long range weapons'. But what happened was that the Bad Wolf side of the 'guards' was *given permission* to engage in its worst possible behaviour. Their Good Wolf was thus switched off by the 'social environment'.

A similar result was found in the Milgram experiments, which were conducted in 1975, by ordinary American citizens chosen right off the streets of New York. They were instructed to electrocute a 'student' who was in a separate room, every time he got an answer wrong on a particular test. The (individual) research participant, playing the role of 'teacher' (in the presence of a supervisor [the researcher]) would read out a question into a microphone. The 'student' (who was collaborating with the researcher) was primed to 'get it wrong', and the 'teacher' was instructed (by the 'supervisor', who was the researcher) to administer greater and greater voltages of electrical shocks to the 'student', who would cry out loudly in (convincing but mock) pain. But despite these pleas to 'stop; I can't go on', the 'teachers' would continue to electrocute the 'student' when told to do so by the research supervisor (in a white lab coat). This showed quite clearly that, while the Bad Wolf in every human can be controlled by an internalized 'inhibitor' – a cultural 'superego', or 'over-I' – normally the voices of mother and father and early school teachers – this superego can be *switched off* by a Bad External Superego in the present moment – such as Zimbardo and Milgram, in their experiments; and senior US army officers in the case of the Mai Lai massacre and the Abu Ghraib prison torture scandal in Iraq (Zimbardo, 2007).

And today, on the streets of Britain, we hear of cases of young men being kicked to death by drunken 'enemies', while they lie on a pavement begging for mercy.

Lorenz's (1966/2002) argument (inferred from animal research) will not stand up in the face of this very convincing counter evidence from research with humans. Of course, Lorenz did eventually go on to acknowledge the importance of moral education in restraining destructive forms of aggression, but by then it was too late. He had effectively denied an innate basis to human badness, or innate evil.

The way in which nature and nurture interact in shaping anger and aggression in individual humans will be explored further in the section of E-CENT, below.

~~~

Chapter 7: Attachment relationships, anger and emotional self-management

"In the right circumstances, there is nothing wrong with anger. Anger is an essential tool for survival. We are programmed to feel anger so that we can deal with threats to our well-being. The physical characteristics of this powerful emotion are designed to enable us to deal with danger, sending signals that our bodies and minds are roused to take action. The anger response is natural and necessary. There is nothing wrong with healthy anger, that is, anger which is based on sound beliefs and is expressed appropriately". Hartley (2002)[47].

~~~

Dr John Bowlby and anger

Dr John Bowlby, the father of attachment theory, studied anger as well as other emotions in families. For example he looks at *angry jealousy* between members of a family, and not just between lovers; and angry outbursts by parents when children take risks with their health and life, as in running across roads – in which cases the anger is mixed with, and perhaps covers over, the initial anxiety. "In the situations described anger is often functional" he says. "When child or spouse behaves dangerously, an angry protest is likely to deter. When a lover's partner strays, a sharp reminder of how much he or she cares may work wonders. When a child finds himself relatively neglected in favour of the new baby, assertion of his claims may redress the balance. Thus in the right place, at the right time, and in right degree, anger is not only appropriate but may be indispensable". (Bowlby, 1988/2005, page 88-89)[48].

Attachment theory and anger management

Dr Daniel Sonkin (2011) has reviewed Attachment theory to see what it can tell us about how to develop anger management processes that are adequate to the task[49]. Those processes must take account of the fact that "Not only do the causes of <u>anger dysregulation</u> differ from person to person, but *the pathways to change will be different* as well". (Page 2)

Dr Sonkin reminds us that Dr John Bowlby – the father of Attachment theory – observed the links and connections between attachment (between mothers and children) and anger (between them) back in the 1930's and 40's:

"John Bowlby first witnessed the effects of infants separated from their mothers in a hospital setting, when intense displays of anger were followed by despair and detachment". (Page 2).

Indeed Bowlby, and other later attachment theorists, argue that it is precisely in our family relationships, or our substitute family relationships, that we learn how to deploy our innate emotions. Bowlby (1988)[50] presents the following description of the relation of emotion to family relationships:

"A feature of attachment behaviour of the greatest importance clinically, and present irrespective of the age of the individual concerned, is the intensity of the emotion that accompanies it, the kind of emotion aroused depending on how the relationship between the individual and the attachment figure is faring. If it goes well, there is joy and a sense of security. If it is threatened, there is jealousy, anxiety, and anger. If broken, there is grief and depression. Finally, there is strong evidence that how attachment behaviour comes to be organized within an individual turns in high degree on the kinds of experience he has in his family of origin, or, if he is unlucky, out of it". (Page 4).

See Bowlby (1988) for more detail.

~~~

Anger as 'calling to mother' to come back

Bowlby's view was that the anger by the child functioned as a signal to the mother/caregiver "…to become available to provide comfort and support, soothing the fear and anxiety associated with separation, at a time when self-soothing capacities are not yet developed". (Sonkin, page 2). This came to be known as the process of "affect regulation" via "limbic resonance". The mother and child communicate in direct emotional ways, and the mother calms the child down and reassures it that all is well in the world, or that at least she understands what is going wrong, and she can put it right. The child is wired up by nature to seek an attachment figure – usually the mother – which will not only ensure its survival, but which will also soothe its central nervous system when it displays negative affects (or emotions). (See:

Lewis, Amini and Lannon, 2001[51]; Gerhardt, 2004[52]; Wallin, 2007[53]; Fonagy and others, 2002[54]; and Schore, 2003[55]).

If the mother/carer is "good enough", then the child will almost certainly receive sufficient sensitive care (and lack of intrusive over-handling) and the child will become emotionally well adjusted – "securely attached" – and gradually, over a period of many years, take back from the parent more and more of their own emotional affect regulation (but never all of it!): (Lewis et al, 2001; and Gerhardt, 2004).

If the mother/carer is not "good enough", then the child will almost certainly receive inadequate responses to its cries for help; inappropriate, or intrusive, or neglectful treatment, which will produce emotional maladjustment – "insecure attachment" – in which case they will fail to learn adequate forms and levels of emotional self-regulation. They may become inhibited sulkers (by developing the "avoidant attachment style"); or they may act out their aggressive feelings in destructive ways (as in the "ambivalent/resistant attachment style"); or they may flip around from being passively angry to aggressively angry, including the possibility of hurting themselves or others (which is the "disorganized attachment style").

The interesting thing about attachment style (and its emotional coping strategies) is that "more often than not", and perhaps in about 75-80% of cases, this relationship style is carried into adulthood. (Sonkin, page 4; Wallin, 2007, pages 37-39).

And not only is it carried into adulthood, but it is also passed down the generations. However, Fonagy (2001) suggests that the research studies are more mixed than implied by others, with some studies providing strong support for intergenerational transmission of attachment styles, and some providing weak support, and some providing no support at all[56]. This contradicts the findings of Mary Main, cited in Wallin (2007, page 37); and this conflict suggests the need for further research on this subject.

Secure attachment keeps us emotionally stable

However, having stated his reservations, Fonagy (2001) goes on to state that:

"There is general agreement that attachment security can serve as a protective factor against psychopathology (or tendency towards emotional distress), and that it is associated with a wide range of healthier personality variables such as lower anxiety (Collins and Read, 1990)[57], less hostility, and greater ego resilience (Kobak and Sceery, 1988)[58], and greater ability to regulate affect – or control our emotions - through interpersonal relatedness (Simpson et al, 1992[59], Valliant 1992[60]).

Insecure attachment appears to be a risk factor and is associated with such characteristics as a greater degree of depression (Armsden and Greenberg 1987a[61]), anxiety, hostility and psychosomatic illness (Hazan and Shaver 1990[62]) and less ego resilience (Kobak and Sceery 1988)". (Fonagy 2001, page 33).

Therefore, although Sonkin's claim is probably too strong – when he states that "This means that strategies for dealing with anger are likely to persist into adulthood" - there are still very good reasons to recommend that stress management coaches and counsellors ask their clients to check their attachment style online, (e.g. at this website:
), and to compare their attachment style with:

(1) their reported style of dealing with anger, and

(2) with the predictions given below (in 'Patterns of anger related to attachment').

One reason that adult attachment style may deviate from childhood attachment style is the concept of "earned security", or "earned secure attachment", whereby an individual becomes more securely attachment to a person outside their family, or within their extended family; or they may find their romantic relationships, or a marriage, to have curative effects upon insecure attachment. (Wallin, 2007, page 87)

Sonkin (2011) presents an interesting list of common patterns of anger, linked to attachment styles:

Patterns of anger related to attachment:

"Based on attachment theory, anger problems can potentially have three possible aetiologies" (or sources/origins):

1: "**Deactivating strategies** (referred to as 'dismissing attachment' in [avoidant] adults[63]) can result in the *passive expression* of anger, being critical and devaluing others, and periodic explosions when holding back is no longer a viable option".

2: "**Hyper-activating strategies** (referred to as 'preoccupied attachment' in [anxious/ambivalent] adults[64]) can result in chronic expression of irritation, anger, and anxiety; hypersensitivity to separation and difference, the chronic blaming of others for the person's distress, attempting to get others to change in order to reduce their anger and anxiety, and difficulty being soothed by others' attempts at caregiving". And, thirdly:

3: "**Disorganized strategies** (referred to as 'unresolved' or 'disorganized' attachment in adults [who had frightening or frightened parents]) can result in extreme expressions of anger that manifest in the inconsistent expression of approach and avoidance strategies, aggression and violence towards self and/or others, dissociation, and PTSD symptomology due to unresolved childhood trauma". (Sonkin, page 5).

Three approaches to anger management

Looking at anger management through this tripartite prism, or lens, gives rise to three different approaches to helping clients manage their anger more constructively[65]. In the presentation that follows, I will deploy some of Sonkin's ideas, plus some of my own.

A person with the 'deactivating style' (#1 above), which is an 'avoidant style' of attachment/relating, will benefit from help with:

(a) "Identifying (their) emotional reactions"; labelling them; defining them; identifying less exaggerated and more verbal ways of responding to the same stimulus; and:

(b) "…learning to make use of dyadic soothing strategies (e.g. seek support from others and talk about their feelings"); and:

(c) Giving up sulking, and replacing it with honest communication, as in the use of reasonable self-assertion.

A person with the 'hyper-activating pattern' (#2 above), which is a form of 'angry clinging', or trying to force compliance, will benefit from help with:

(a) "…containing their emotional reactivity while learning to develop more self-soothing strategies (which involves depending more on self during times of distress).

(b) Learning to 'stand in love' rather than 'fall in love'. To stand on their own two feet. To learn that they are capable of independent living; surviving without constant contact with or support from others.

(c) Learning to transfer their (adult) attachment from one individual to the idea that they are a part of the whole universe. There is nowhere to fall to, because we are each glued into the web of life.

A person with the 'disorganized pattern' (#3 above), which sometimes presents as psychotic or 'personality disordered' behaviour, will benefit from help to:

(a) "…resolve trauma and loss that contributes to intense emotional states that result in a collapse of coping strategies that can lead to harming others and oneself". (Sonkin, page 5).

(b) Reassurance that the world is not as frightening as it may have seemed in their childhood.

(c) Help to complete any grief work that has been left incomplete from childhood onwards.

From this review of Attachment theory in relation to anger, we can see that there are no simple solutions to anger management, and we need to take great care in attempting to understand the source of a person's anger, and the best solution for them individually.

~~~

Chapter 8: The neurobiological perspective

> '"There is no longer any doubt" writes Kandel, "that psychotherapy can result in detectable changes in the brain". Recent brain scans done before and after psychotherapy show both that the brain plastically reorganizes itself in treatment and that the more successful the treatment the greater the change.' Doidge (2008), Page 233[66].

Introduction

Because emotions occur within the human body-brain-mind, they have been difficult to understand by philosophers and psychologists in the past.

In recent times, the challenge of understanding emotions, like anger, has been greatly helped by the development of new equipment and experiments in neurobiology.

Joseph LeDoux and Antonio Damasio are prominent among these new theorists of the mind and emotions.

More recent theorists include: Jaak Panksepp, Allan Schore, and Daniel Siegel.

Three approaches to emotion research

There are three common approaches to emotion research:

1. The basic emotions approach, which asserts that we can construct lists of the basic emotions that are innate in humans (anger being one of those basic emotions);

2. The component-additive approach, in which we do not use basic emotions, but combine them into complex emotions. We learn how to combine emotions and body actions in early life; for example by learning to combine visceral[67], autonomic and bodily components, like tensing the body and furrowing the brow when angry about frustration; baring the lower teeth and scowling at an adversary; etc.

And:

3. The social constructionist approach, which says emotions are social constructs (or emotions are co-constructed in our earliest relationships). We learn how to emote from our family of origin.

The E-CENT perspective is that none of these theories is correct in itself, but that, sensibly combined, they begin to provide a reasonable explanation of emotions.

Sonkin (2011) reminds us that Antonio Damasio provides five axioms for clarifying the nature of emotions, and I will review those axioms now:

1. Emotions are complex aggregations of chemical and neural responses to environmental stimulation that are involved in the management of moment to moment life.

A baby has an innate set of primitive emotions, which have developmental capabilities, provided they are met by a social environment that supports and interacts with the new baby. Those innate primitive emotions are located in the brain stem, the limbic system, and in the viscera of the chest and belly. They are also linked to the facial muscles and other parts of the body through the central nervous system. Those emotions are designed by nature to ensure the survival of the new baby. If the baby did not become angrily distressed when hungry, it might die of malnourishment.

2. As the baby develops, its cultural learning will alter the expression of its emotions and give them new meanings. Nevertheless, emotions are biologically determined processes that have evolved over time.

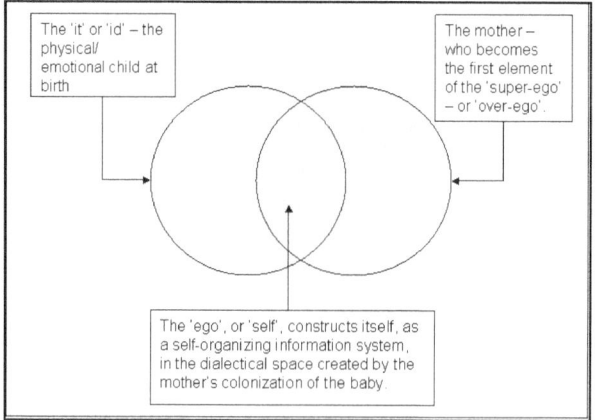

Figure 8.1: The most basic model of E-CENT theory:

The dialectical nature of the individual/social ego.

The message of Figure 8.1 above is this: The ego is a product of relationship, and cannot exist without (external and/or internalized) relationship.

The innate emotions in the 'it', or the child at birth (shown by the left-hand circle), are designed by nature to (eventually, developmentally) provide the basis of the fight/flee/freeze response, and other basic biological responses of seeking attachment (love) and seeking autonomy (curiosity, rebellion against control, etc.) At birth the child can show pleasure and displeasure, and those shows of displeasure are embryonic anger responses.

The socially shaped emotions in the mother are a result of her socialization by her mother, and her wider education by her culture. She has learned to have a particular attitude towards anger – to express it, or to hide it, to fear it, and so on.

As the mother and baby interact, they braid together in the ego space (the central, overlapping, dialectical space of the two circles [of Fig 8.1]) - producing a fusion of the baby's innate biologically determined emotions, and the mother's socially shaped emotions, to produce the baby's own socially shaped emotions.

3. The parts of the brain that produce emotions occupy a fairly restricted ensemble of subcortical regions, beginning at the level of the brain stem and moving up to the higher brain.

The innate, biologically determined emotions are contained in the lower brain regions, and those in the limbic system can be modified by experience. In addition, emotionalized experiences are stored in the neocortex, and those memories of historical emotion-events also play a key part in the generation of emotional responses. So an individual who grows up in an angry family will have different memories to draw upon than an individual who grows up within a more peaceful, calm family. And so, their innate anger expressions will also differ.

4. All emotions can and do operate unconsciously, and it's only when we are <u>aware</u> of having an emotion (in the form of a mental representation) that we are <u>having a feeling</u> (or an emotional affect).

Human beings are creatures of habit, who operate mainly tacitly from non-conscious levels of mind. This applies as much to emotional responses as it does to spoken and physical responses. When a person responds angrily, they are enacting a non-consciously stored habit, applied to a context by an association or similarity. To become non-angry in these anger-inducing contexts, an 'angry individual' must learn a new set of habits, and form new associations between environmental stimuli and responses.

5. All emotions are experienced in the body. But they also affect the brain-mind as well.

This is a drift back towards the James-Lange theory of emotion, which we do not accept in E-CENT. Our model is as follows:

The James-Lange theory says that emotions begin in the body, during each emotion-experience; so that the body is the primary source of emotions. We disagree with this view. We see the mind and body as both being equally involved in emotion responses. That is to say, emotions occur in the body-brain-mind.

Of course, it could be objected that Walter Cannon put a major fly in my ointment with his experiments which seemed to show that an experimental animal surgically separated from its viscera, could still feel fear. However, Cannon and Bard's theory does not cause me much concern. They considered "...the physiological changes to be a sort of side effect - useful in preparing the body to take appropriate action but not essential to our conscious experience of emotion". (Kagan and Segal, 1992, page 324).

My own view is closer to that of Nicolas Humphrey (1992), who got around the problem of Cannon and Bard's reservations by working on the mystery of *phantom limb syndrome*. An individual who has lost his hand may occasionally feel strong sensations in the "missing hand", and want to scratch it. This phenomenon goes on for many years after the hand was lost, and possibly for the remainder of the individual's life.

Humphrey (1992) resolved this conundrum by realizing that, through a process of evolution, an original system of sending a signal from body surface to brain, and a response back to the original part of the body surface, the brain had learned to create brain-based representations of the source of the stimulus, and to maintain two loops. The first, a long one, runs from the body surface to the brain and back again, while the second, a short one, runs from the sensing part of the brain, to the brain-based representation of that part of the body. Thus a person may have a missing hand, but they still have *a brain-based representation of that hand*, which can "feel" sensations (possibly in the motor cortex, or a related site). By corollary, it is my contention that the brain contains stored representations of what it was like - (at Y - some level of physiological arousal) - to be anxiously aroused, angrily aroused and so on. This is crudely represented in Figure 8.2:

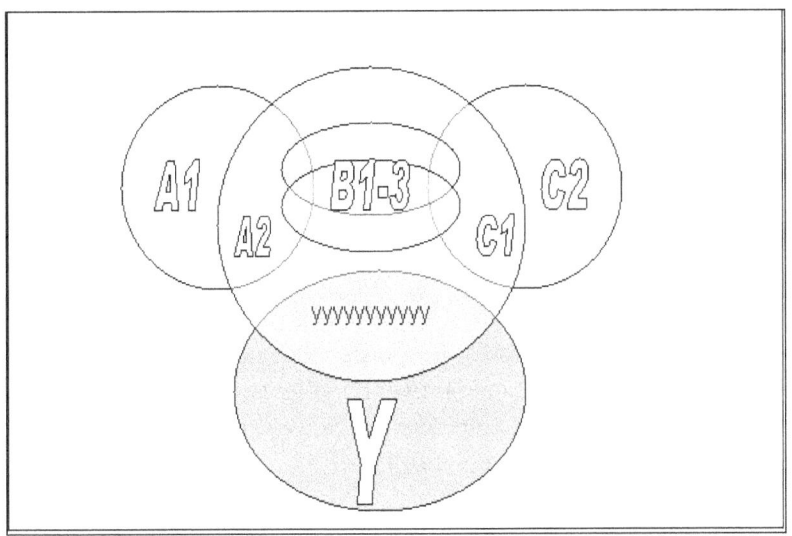

Figure 8.2 - The A>B>Y>y>C Model al la Humphrey-Byrne Linkages

Figure 8.2 shows the body as the grey ellipse (Y); and the head/brain/mind as the large circle in the middle of the frame. Using the model in Figure 8.2, we would say that a stimulus at A1 (which is an 'event' or 'object' outside the person) triggers a percept (in the form of an interpretive inference at A2), which triggers an evaluative (cognitive-emotive) processing of that signal at B1-3 (which are the three components of the overlapping of cognitive and emotive processing centres [in the orbitofrontal cortex [OFC]).

The B1 or 2 or 3 (discussed fully in Byrne, 2017) then sends out *at least* three signals. One goes to the face-body to initiate a physiological response. One goes to the collection of little internal y's, (inside the B boundary – in the brain/mind/body) representing physiological responses to previous stimuli of the type apprehended at A2 (and now stored in long-term memory). And one goes straight to the C1 to signal an affective output. The brain-based little y's yield up the best fit to A2 of *historically appropriate* physiological arousal, and send a signal to C1 containing that information. (This is similar to what is called 'pattern matching' in the 'Human Givens' tradition: Griffin and Tyrrell, 2004[68]). It is anticipated that the signal from B1/2/3 and the signal from the little internal Y's will meet and combine at C1, and initiate (and sometimes modify) the affective output at C2. Perhaps one second later, the feedback signal from the bodily Y will reach C1, and reinforce the output at C2. And the *hormonal responses*, running *behind* the electrical signals, will further reinforce that message, perhaps another second later.

All of these processes are governed by the fundamental principle that the organism, including the human organism, is a creature of *habit*, and outputs are selected on the basis of best fit from a relatively limited collection of *historically accumulated representations* in long term memory. Habitual ways of responding may be broken *after reflection* upon them, but *not* in the process of responding to a new stimulus. (This was the only truth in the old behaviourist theory of Stimulus>Response>No Choice! Free will in humans is mainly "Free won't - after the event!" We can dispute our 'irrational beliefs', or 'unreasonable preferences', once we find out what they are, but we *cannot* eliminate them in advance!)

So, therefore, angry thoughts, angry feelings and angry actions go hand in hand. To eliminate one, we have to tackle all three. And we have to work on the body sources of anger as much as the mind sources. Thus diet, exercise and sleep – which all affect brain health – are as important as self-talk and philosophy of life. And historical and current relationships, and our attachments styles, also play their roles in determining our patterns of anger.

~~~

Chapter 9: The Stoic perspective on anger

The philosophy of Stoicism has much to teach us about anger, especially Seneca's essay 'On Anger'.[69] But Stoicism has strengths *and weaknesses* in its explanation of anger.

Moderate Stoicism is an empowering philosophy of life – including a system of logic and a unique cosmology, combined with a *compensatory philosophy* for coping with the undoubted difficulties of life. The cosmology of Stoicism does not contain a transcendent deity, or god/gods, but rather it posits an indwelling rational principle of a 'fiery substance' of which each of our souls is seen to be a part. (Aurelius, 1992[70]; Epictetus, 1991[71]; Irvine, 2009[72].)

Stoicism was created by Zeno of Citium, in ancient Greece, about 300 BCE[73]. Zeno had studied Cynicism with Crates, plus some of Plato's philosophy at the Academy (Irvine, 2009, pages 32-33). His own life had been seriously disadvantaged by a shipwreck at sea, in which he lost all his material assets, and his philosophy partly constitutes a coming to terms with the harshness of life as he experienced it. Stoicism survived for at least 400 years, in Greece, and, in slightly modified form, in ancient Rome.

According to the Stoic view of life, anger is one of the 'passions'. Seddon (2000)[74] tells us that: "In Stoic theory there are four primary passions:

- **desire** … is an impulse towards some anticipated thing regarded as good;

- **fear** … is an impulse away from some anticipated things regarded as bad.

The other two (passions) are:

- **delight** …, an impulse towards some present thing regarded as good, and

- **distress** …, an impulse away from some present thing regarded as bad…

Anger, sexual desire and love of riches for instances, are types of **desire** …

The Stoics explain the passions in terms of the judgements we make regarding the circumstances we find ourselves in". (Seddon, 2000, page 2).

This taxonomy of passions has its appeal, and it seems in many respects to be intuitively right. However, it is probably better to see *anger as a **response** to the blocking of some important desire*, rather than an *expression* of a desire. (In E-CENT, we see *inappropriate anger* as being pretty central to the emotional state called the Bad Wolf. While the Good Wolf is driven by love, and *appropriate* anger; the Bad Wolf is driven by hatred, and *inappropriate* anger).

However, when we assert our reasonable rights as an equal individual, in a democratic society, we have to use *some degree of healthy anger*. But it seems that, for a Stoic, all anger is bad anger. We do not accept this extreme position; while we do accept the Stoic view that anger (or rather, [I would add] *unhealthy* anger) causes a lot of major problems in the world:

"Anger, says Seneca, is 'brief insanity' and the damage done by anger is enormous: 'No plague has cost the human race more'. Because of anger, he says, we see all around us people being killed, poisoned and sued; we see cities and nations ruined. And besides destroying cities and nations, anger can destroy us individually. We live in a world, after all, in which there is much to be angry about, meaning that unless we can learn to control our anger, we will be perpetually angry. Being angry, Seneca concludes, is a waste of precious time". (Irvine, 2009: page 159).

We agree that excessive, rageful anger causes all the problems above; and so it is important to give up rageful, excessive anger. But you need to keep your reasonable, assertive anger, which fuels you determination to ask for what you want, to say no to what you do not want, and to engage *constructive* confrontation! (*Ask* for what you want. Or, *say no* to what you do not want. Or say: "When you do X, I feel Y, because..." And when the other person responds in a volatile or angry manner, just reflect what they are saying, or the feelings they are displaying, until they calm down. The resend you assertive message: "When you do X, I feel Y, because..." Keep going until they agree to make changes to how they have treated you, about which you are assertively complaining!)

~~~

Returning to the Stoic perspective, anger for a Stoic is a *passion*, induced by a *judgement* that something bad is being done to us, and we have to retaliate:

According to Seddon (2000): "…the passions have an essential cognitive (or thinking) component without which they would not be able to serve, as they do, as ways for us to relate to what goes on in the world. Passions are grounded in *how we find the world*, in how we *judge matters*; this being so, the passions can be evaluated as appropriate or inappropriate, justified or unjustified". (Seddon, 2000, page 3).

This is what Epictetus meant, in the Enchiridion, when he said: "(Wo)men are disturbed not by the things which happen, but by the opinions[75] about the things. … When, then, we are impeded or disturbed or grieved, let us never blame others, but ourselves, that is, our opinions". (The *Enchiridion*, page 14).

We do not accept this *extreme perspective* in E-CENT.

Why not?

Because, if I become angry when a man punches me in the face, I am angry…

(A) Because of the punch; and:

(B) The precise intensity of my anger is a result of the nature of my opinion (judgement). (But also, my impulse control is affected by whether or not I had a good night's sleep last night; and whether or not I have recently eaten junk foods containing trans-fats! And whether or not I have recently done enough physical exercise to burn off, and thus reduce, my stress hormones).

I am angry because of the punch in the same way that any animal will respond with *fight* or *flight* (or freeze) if you strike it. And my response will be based on my habitual way of dealing with such assaults; which, in turn, will have been *socially shaped by a whole range of experiences*, with mother and father (when I was a baby!), siblings, local peers, school peers, and so on. Cognitively, my *expectations* also play a role. But it is wrong of Seddon (2000) to imply that there is a 'thinking component', if by 'thinking component' he means a *conscious* thought, in words. And it is also wrong if he is saying that my thoughts are separate from my feelings. In fact, my so-called thoughts are underpinned by my capacity to make emotive evaluations of my experiences.

So the correct equation here is this:

The incoming stimulus (S), is processed by me as a whole organism (O), and I output a response (in this case anger) on the basis of my general state of being, including my habitual way of dealing with such an assault, and my current state of body-brain-mind, based on my diet, exercise, sleep, and general stress level, etc.

I can reduce the intensity of my anger by working on my diet, exercise, sleep hygiene, philosophy of life, and my general stress level.

In fact, to the degree that it is possible to infer that I have language-based thoughts about anger-inducing stimuli, then I may be said to have *two attitudes* towards the possibility that you might punch me.

- The first is a 'moral must': *"You (morally) must not, ought not to punch me"*.

- The second is a 'strong preference': *"I do not want you (or anybody else) to ever punch me, and I will do whatever I can do avoid this happening, including physically defending myself"*.

E-CENT does not blame the individual's opinions/judgements/beliefs for their emotional distress. We take reality into account also. We modify Epictetus by saying: "People *are* upset by the negative things that happen to them, but the intensity of their upset is a function of their *habitual expectations/beliefs/attitudes/opinions/judgements* towards the things that happen to them (all of which is affected by historical experience, current stressors, and diet, exercise, sleep, etc."

Thus an individual can reduce their passion from 'anger' to 'mild irritation or annoyance', by changing their body-brain-mind along the lines indicated in the previous paragraph.

But Stoic philosophy was created in an era – two thousand years ago, and more, when psychology did not exist; neuroscience did not exist; nutritional and exercise science did not exist; stress management theory did not exist; and so on.

Seddon (2000) goes on to say, in effect, that the Stoics believed that the passion of anger is a result of anger-inducing judgements (which, I have argued, is a gross over-simplification of the multi-causes of anger):

"An *evaluation* that we have been slighted, for example, *justifies* (to us) and makes sense of our angry response. My feeling angry, and my displaying anger, only makes sense in a context where *I believe* (whether I really have reason to or not) that I have been treated unjustly, have been taken advantage of, insulted or something of the sort". (Seddon, 2000, page 3).

This is Epictetus' theory in practice. He claims that we are *unaffected* by external reality. For Epictetus and Seddon, anger is a result of an *inaccurate evaluation* of personal harm. According to Epictetus and Marcus Aurelius, *nobody can harm us*, because 'harm' mean 'denying us the possibility of acting on our own values and virtues'. But this is not an accurate definition of *harm*, in the context of humans having fleshy bodies, which can be pierced, bruised, burned, crushed, and killed. The human body-brain-mind has survived for more than 200,000 years, and our (easily angered) primate ancestors may go back more than two million years. None of those generations of primate and human body-minds would have been likely to survive, in the presence of many predators, if we did not have a powerful *physical-kinaesthetic urge* to remain alive against all odds (which is manifested in *the totally automatic fight or flight response of the sympathetic nervous system!*

I think it was George Bernard Shaw who said that anybody who can support the cited statement by Epictetus – that we are unaffected by what happens to us, and that nothing can harm us, except by denying us the possibility of acting on our own chosen virtues - obviously *has never spent an hour walking naked into a freezing blizzard!*

If we agree that a noxious stimulus is normally present before a passion of anger appears, we also have to concede that the 'noxious activating events' in our lives play *some role* in promoting anger. ***People do not normally make themselves angry unless there is some ostensible or actual negative event which at least*** <u>***seems to them***</u> ***(instinctively, automatically, non-thinkingly) to impact their lives negatively!***

And "seeming to them" does not just depend upon their *opinions*, in their *heads*; but also on their recent experience of *sleep* (adequate or inadequate); *blood sugar level*, resulting from recent (sufficiency or insufficiency) of healthy food; stress level (which is related to physical exercise, and social-environmental pressures, etc.), at home and in work, and in the wider world!

The core of the liberational effect of Stoicism is expressed by Seddon (2000) as follows:

"…Passions (like anger) can always be avoided by deciding to withhold our assent to the effect that anything really good or really bad is happening to us. If I do not judge that I have been slighted, I will not be angry..." (Ibid, page 3).

While this statement is technically true, it is often impossible for mere mortals to agree that they have not been slighted, when, for example, they have been unfairly dismissed; and denied the right to manage their own environment. How do I know this is true? Because this is what happened to Dr Albert Ellis, who spent fifty years trying to train his counselling clients, his students, his colleagues and the readers of his books, that they can avoid anger by changing their beliefs about noxious activating events, like slights, insults, and deprivations, etc. But when it happened to him, in 2004-2005, he did get angry; and he did sue his former colleagues for unfair dismissal; thus demonstrating that, while it is easy to *talk the talk* of Extreme Stoicism, it is often impossible to *walk the walk*!

The trick performed by Extreme Stoics is this: They change the meaning of 'good' and 'bad' _from their conventional use_, and indeed only consider virtue and virtuous acts to be good. (Everything else, they say, is 'indifferent'). And they hold that only their own vices and vicious acts are actually bad. This will obviously work – for committed Stoics - as a way of *reframing* the nature of reality, but it is more than a bit of a stretch for most people. Most people (including the Arch Stoic, Albert Ellis) will fall at the first hurdle!

Because the Stoic definition of 'bad' is so far from conventional usage, we in E-CENT do not use this definition. We still encourage our clients to reframe their noxious activating events, but in a different way. It could be said that we use a 'different level' of reframing; one that comes from Moderate Buddhism and Moderate Stoicism – while rejecting the extremes of both of these philosophies. (For an example of extremism: a Good Zen Buddhist is supposed to be so *unattached to life* that, if instructed by their 'master' to commit hara-kiri [which is suicide by slitting their stomach with a sharp sword] they would not hesitate to follow that instruction! And extreme Stoicism has some equally unappealing 'commitments').

In our E-CENT approach, we **grant** that something which has happened to you *may genuinely be bad*, such as losing your job, or your home, or being insulted or snubbed. We do not ask you to agree that these events are *not bad*. And we certainly do not describe them as "indifferent" acts or events. Instead we ask you to look at them through a range of 'windows', or 'frames', or lenses including the following:

1. Life is difficult (frustrating and somewhat painful) for **all humans**, much of the time. Therefore, it is obviously going to be difficult for you; at least some of the time. Do not make the mistake of insisting that your life should be without any difficulty whatsoever!)

2. Life would not seem so bad or difficult if we could avoid 'picking' and 'choosing' altogether. But this is difficult for most humans. So reduce your 'pickings and choosings' to reasonable, modest levels. If you feel very upset about losing or failing; or being shunned by somebody, you are probably 'choosing' that "this is too difficult to have happened me!" However, since life is difficult for all human beings, why would you think that you should not have to face your fair share of problems? Surely it is obvious that, (logically and practically), it should be the way it is.[76]

There are an additional four Windows in the basic E-CENT model. (See Byrne, 2018; Chapter 6)[77].

We do agree with the (moderate) Stoic view that acting from virtue is the highest good for a human – and for a human community. We also agree that acting out a vice – or acting viciously, immorally – is the greatest badness a human can do.

However unlike the Stoics, we see many other things as good and bad. It's bad to live near a noisy motorway, because of the negative health impact of the noise and the fumes. And it is good to live in a place with fresh air and fresh water, in a quiet, harmonious community. Because some of these things are good for us and some of them are bad for us, it is preferable to get the good things and preferable to avoid the bad things. These cannot be treated as matters of supreme *indifference!*

If we act from virtue, avoid vice, and stick to preferring that we mainly get those secondary goods, and avoid the secondary badness, we will mainly avoid anger. (Unless we eat junk foods containing trans-fats; have sleep disturbance or sleep deprivation; fail to do an adequate amount of physical exercise, and so on).

We will not anger ourselves, in the context described in the previous paragraph, because *inappropriate anger is the core of our 'bad side'* (which we in E-CENT call our 'Bad Wolf'). We will not anger ourselves when we fail to acquire secondary goods, because *we only prefer them*, and therefore we will not disturb ourselves (and certainly not *anger ourselves*) about not getting them. (It would be nice, but we do not have to get what is nice!)

E-CENT theory agrees with the (moderate) Stoic view that we should be *fatalistic* about the *past* and the *present moment*, and only have goals for *the future*[78]. We therefore *cannot (inappropriately) anger ourselves* about any frustrations or insults from the past or the present moment.

If somebody close to us frustrates or insults us, we should assert ourselves about our concerns about *their future behaviour* towards us. And we must forgive them their past transgressions – provided they do not continue to treat us badly. (If they continue to treat us badly, we should *seriously consider* decamping to a more congenial environment!)

And our goals for the future should not be about becoming wealthy or famous, since we cannot control such outcomes. Instead, we would be well advised to set goals which involve preferring that we acquire some secondary goods (such as good health, happiness, successful relationships, and particular career outcomes, etc.); and preferring to avoid some secondary bad outcomes (such as the effects of alcohol, junk food, pharmaceutical drugs, bad relationships, exploitative employment, and so on). The goals that are likely to make us happiest involve making a contribution to our family, community, work, and to other individuals (Irvine, 2009; and Ben-Shahar, 2007)[79].

We question the Stoic goal of striving to perfect our rational and virtuous sides, and to shrink our irrational and vicious sides. Why?

Because we see this as *a muddled classification* of aspects of the brain-mind.

Our rational functioning (perceiving-thinking-reasoning) depends upon our irrational-emotional side, without which we would not be able to evaluate or value anything. (Damasio, 1994, 2000).

For us, the *rational* cannot be equated with the *virtuous*, since we need the moral emotions (or *irrationals*) of *guilt* and *shame,* and *emotional empathy*, in order to fuel our so called 'reasoning' about moral issues.

We have an innate capacity to be both moral and immoral – and those capacities are *fuelled by irrational (non-reasoning) tendencies*. But through the process of *socialized moral teachings,* we elaborate our approach to virtue and vice. The more you grow your 'good side' (which I call the Good Wolf), and shrink your Bad Wolf, the less you will be likely to respond angrily to anybody or anything.

And always remember, the rational side of a human being (the 'Adult ego state', in Transactional Analysis [TA]) is split down the middle between Goodness and Badness. For an illustration, imagine an intelligent man (or woman) who works overtime on the refinement of their rational skill, in order to find a fool-proof way to break into the local bank and take all the money that's stored there!

~~~

To grow your Good Wolf, you need to pay attention to the balance of good and bad actions in your daily behaviour. This is what Epictetus meant when he said: "(The Stoic philosopher) … watches him/herself as if s/he were an enemy and lying in ambush"[80]. The enemy within is the Bad Wolf.

If you are going to watch yourself in this way, to ensure that you are not engaging in immoral opinions or judgements that are making you unnecessarily angry, then one way to proceed is to have a journal and to write in it at the end of each day: To examine your conscience; to assess your performance; to evaluate your behaviours towards others. This is a process that a number of prominent Stoics have used over the years, as described by Irvine (2009; Chapter 8) and Seddon (2000). Here's Seddon's description:

"All our senses ought to be trained to endurance. They are naturally long-suffering (or strong and resilient), if only the mind desists from weakening them. This (mind) should be summoned to give an account of itself every day. Sextius had this habit, and when the day was over and he had retired to his nightly rest, he would put these questions to his soul (or mind):

'What bad habit have you cured today? What fault have you resisted? In what respect are you better?'

"Anger will cease and become more controllable if it finds that it must appear before a judge every day. Can anything be more excellent than this practice of thoroughly sifting the whole day? And how delightful the sleep that follows this self-examination – how tranquil it is, how deep and untroubled, when the soul (or mind) has either praised or admonished itself, and when this secret examiner and critic of self has given report of its own character! I avail myself of this privilege, and every day I plead my cause before the bar of self. When the light has been removed from sight, and my wife, long aware of my habit, has become silent, I scan the whole of my day and retrace all my deeds and words. I conceal nothing from myself, I omit nothing. For why should I shrink from any of my mistakes, when I may commune thus with myself?"

Seneca then gives some examples of the way he judges the actions he is reviewing, at the end of the day; and how he speaks to himself about them:

'See that you never do that again; I will pardon you this time. In that dispute, you spoke too offensively; after this don't have encounters with ignorant people; those who have never learned do not want to learn. You reproved that (wo)man more frankly than you ought, and consequently you have not so much mended him/her as offended him/her. In the future, consider not only the truth of what you say, but also whether the (wo)man to whom you are speaking can endure the truth. A good (wo)man accepts reproof gladly; the worse a (wo)man is the more bitterly s/he resents it.' Seneca, quoted in Seddon (2000), pages 6-7.

In the Stoic view, anger is bad for social relationships; but it is primarily bad because it spoils our tranquillity. Tranquilly is the reward for living a good life. Tranquillity is the core of the Stoic form of happiness: *eudaimonia*.

Irvine (2009) relays the following Stoic advice on avoiding anger:

- Don't be so sensitive to feedback from others; toughen yourself up; do not be too attracted to comfort;

- apologise if you express anger towards anybody; use humour to deflect insults; don't take yourself too seriously;

- resist believing the worst about others, and impugning their motives; remember that the things that anger us most often do not do us any real harm; and remember that the people who anger us are also most likely angered by us!

Dr Ed Jacobs would caution this: "Always keep your expectations in line with reality"[81].

And here is a useful take on reality, from Marcus Aurelius:

"Say to yourself in the early morning: I shall meet today inquisitive, ungrateful, violent, treacherous, envious, uncharitable men (and women). All these things have come upon them through ignorance of real good and ill (or evil)".[82]

If you set out with this mindset, why would you quickly or easily anger yourself when somebody blocks your path, insults you, or snubs you; refuses to help you; and in fact hinders you?

You are much less likely to do so. And when you needed to, you would find it much easier to be calm enough to assert your rights with them (fuelled by moderate, appropriate levels of anger, irritation or annoyance).

Thus, your anger would be under reasonable control.

~~~

Get your anger under reasonable control

Chapter 10: The Buddhist perspective on anger

Buddhist philosophy and psychology contain a wealth of useful ideas for anger management. This is so because Buddhism is one of the best understandings of human emotional wiring and thought patterns.

The Four Noble Truths

Gautama (The Buddha) never intended to found a religion. He was primarily interested in how to develop a set of strategies to question our experience, and to live ethically.

The philosophy of the Buddha is based on his 'Four Noble Truths'[83]. These are:

> 1. That life is suffering (Dukkha)[84]. (This is Window No.1 in the E-CENT model).
>
> 2. That suffering has a cause (Desire, or 'Thirst' for life). (This is Window No.2).[85]
>
> 3. A description of how suffering can be ended. And:
>
> 4. A description of the road to the end of suffering.

Using this model, we could say that anger is a form of suffering which arises from desiring that certain things should happen, and certain other things should not happen. But let us look at the matter more deeply.

Transcending the ego and avoiding harm to others

Buddhism is a spiritual practice, or a form of 'mental liberation', aimed at 'transcending everyday reality', and experiencing the peace and tranquility of knowing ourselves to be just a small piece of the total universe; a leaf on the tree of life. (This is part of the road to escaping from suffering).

Buddhists seek to shrink their ego, or sense of self-importance; to act from loving-kindness towards all sentient beings (animals capable of conscious states), and to endure all the difficulties of life by calm acceptance of whatever happens to be the case. They also seek detachment from desiring, as desire is seen as the source of all human suffering.[86]

But Buddhism is not just about a set of attitudes towards the self. In fact, the first of the five precepts that Buddhists adopt is this:

"I undertake the precept to refrain from harming living creatures".[87]

This principle is called 'ahimsā' and it is considerably broader in practice than the practice of avoiding physical harm to another. This is how Keown (2005) describes it:

"Although (ahimsā) literally means 'non-harming' or 'non-violence', it embodies much more than these negative-sounding translations suggest. *Ahimas* is not simply the *absence* of something, but is practiced on the basis of a deeply positive feeling of respect for living beings, a moral position associated in the west with the terms 'respect for life' or 'sanctity of life'." This includes "...concern (dayā) and sympathy (anukampa) for living creatures, and an increasing empathy with them *based on the awareness that others dislike pain and death just as much as oneself"*. (Keown, 2005, page 14).

This is a huge step up from the Stoic perspective, which effectively denies the need for empathy or sympathy or concern for others, by asserting that the difficulties, insults and injuries of life *cannot harm anybody!*

Here are two quotations from Kornfield (1994)[88] which illustrate the depth of *ahimsa*:

"Harm no other beings. They are just your brothers and sisters".

"Like the mother of the world, touch (metaphorically!) each (and every) being as your beloved child"

Anger is the road to hell

However, no matter how 'enlightened' a person may become, through their Buddhist practice, they are always liable to respond angrily if they are seriously thwarted, or frustrated, or insulted/offended. But why do we react like this. One perspective is as follows:

"If we examine how anger or hateful thoughts arise in us, we will find that, generally speaking, they arise when we feel hurt, when we feel that we have been unfairly treated by someone against our expectations. If in that instant we examine carefully the way anger arises, there is a sense that it comes as a protector, comes as a friend that would help our battle, or in taking revenge against the person who has inflicted harm on us. So the anger or hateful thought that arises appears to come as a shield or a protector. But in reality that is an illusion. It is a very delusory state of mind".

In practice we need to stay level-headed; to assess our situation calmly, so that we may respond appropriately. If we succumb to our hottest emotions, we may be acting from an immature part of ourselves. We need to reason out our response. We cannot reliably trust our hottest emotions.

This truth, and the lessons it can teach us, is nicely illustrated in the story of the Samurai warrior seeking teaching from a Zen monk.

"Teach me the truth about heaven and hell", the samurai warrior requested of his Zen teacher.

"What would a stupid great lump like you need with knowledge of heaven and earth?", asked the Zen master with obvious disdain.

The samurai warrior's face flushed. He was enraged. With his face contorted into a mask of hatred, he drew his sword and held it high above the Zen master's head, preparing to slice him in two.

"There", said the Zen master suddenly, smiling, and pointing at the samurai warrior's angry pose. "There is the gate to hell!"

The samurai warrior, instantly enlightened, lowered and dropped his sword, and made a deep bow of gratitude and loving kindness towards his teacher.

"And there", said the Zen master, pointing towards this humble pose: "That is the gate to heaven!"

Defining anger

According to the Buddhist view, anger is one of "the three poisons", because they pollute our tranquil minds, and spoil our sense of peace and detachment from wanting, desiring, grasping. The other two poisons are "greed and ignorance"[89].

Some Buddhist theorists define anger like this:

Anger is

(1) Being **unable to bear** the object (or other person/thing), and

(2) The **intention to cause harm** to the object (or other person/thing).

"Anger is defined as *aversion* with stronger exaggeration".

And *aversion* is defined as: "Exaggerated wanting to be separated from someone or something".[90]

The intention to cause harm must be resisted, for legal and moral reasons, and also out of self-respect. It will not benefit any individual (in any ultimately important respect) to harm another.

And experience shows that actually we <u>can</u> bear the trials and tribulations that life, and other people, throw at us. (Especially if we are well rested, well fed with nourishing food, well watered, and well exercised).

Buddhists do not consider that anger is ever justified, because:

(1) Anger is normally an exaggerated state of arousal about a significantly misinterpreted event, and thus is not accurate; and:

(2) It blocks the sufferer from achieving the transcendent state of tranquil, peaceful mind.

Charlotte Joko Beck, who teaches Zen at the Zen Center, in San Diego, California, tells a little story that puts this in perspective[91]. This is how it goes:

Imagine you are out on a lake in a rowboat, on a very foggy day. You cannot see more than a couple of feet in any direction. Suddenly out of the fog looms another boat, and it's heading straight for your own boat, which you have recently had repainted at great cost. You immediately react with anger towards the 'idiot' who is about to damage your boat, your interests, your personal domain.

Next, you notice that there is nobody in the other boat. The boat is empty. It is drifting under its own momentum across the windblown lake.

Suddenly your anger diminishes, and disappears altogether, because the boat is empty! You reach for a fishing pole, and push the intruding boat out of your path.

What happened here? How do we account for the switch in emotional responses?

You were 'projecting' a 'detestable being' onto the 'pilot' of the boat, and suddenly you realized that there was no 'pilot'! Then your negative projective collapsed, and all you were left with was a practical problem: how to stop the collision of two boats.

Now imagine you are shopping in a city centre, and somebody walks right into you, and up comes your anger. But remember – the boat it empty! The 'boat' of this person is truly empty! There is no conscious 'pilot' managing the trajectory of the body's movements. This person is simply 'drifting across the lake' under its own (non-conscious) momentum. 'The boat is empty' is another way of saying, 'this person – being a human – is sleepwalking right into me'. That's how humans tend to be. Too bad. It would be nice if they were conscious beings who computed every step they take, but they are not. (But there is no malice; not intent to offend me; no *pilot* in the crow's nest!)

The boat is empty!

Stop distressing yourself about the 'malign intent' of empty boats!

Hot, inappropriate anger by definition is about desiring/grasping/greed, and it poisons the mind by introducing hatred and rage at self or others, or at the world.

Of course, I am not advocating that anybody should make themselves a victim of others. But our response should be measured, rational and reasonable. Action against transgressors may be pursued in a non-angry manner, to teach the other person a lesson, or to preserve the rule of law. (Source[92]). Or, as we say in E-CENT, avoid aggressive anger, and simply *assert your reasonable rights* or preferences respectfully.

~~~

Buddhist strategies for defusing anger

Buddhism teaches that we can only defuse anger by developing forgiveness, tolerance, compassion, patience and loving-kindness. (See Chapter 2 on forgiveness).

However, most of us will experience some degree of anger from time to time, and we need strategies to defuse it.

Buddhist mindfulness would encourage us to be aware of all of our thoughts and emotions as they come and go. So when anger arises, observe it, focus on it, and *complete* your experience of it: (especially by 'naming it'! [You've got to name it to tame it, according to Daniel Siegel (2015), the creator of Interpersonal Neurobiology]). This will tend to detach you (the observer) from it, and to shrink it. You also will not be feeding it.

If you are involved in a heated exchange with somebody: Step back. Walk away, counting to ten. Stop. Close your eyes. Imagine a zip fastener down your back, which you can pull down, and step out of your own back. Walk around to the side, so you have a side view of yourself, and imaging the other person is confronting you. *How do you feel as you see this confrontation 'from the outside'? What do you think about it all? What is the solution?*

That set of exercises, in the previous paragraph, will tend to help you to calm down, to think-feel-perceive more constructively about the conflict, and to generate a viable solution which avoids escalation into violence.

Practice daily meditation, so that your mind is calm by habit; and you are in touch with your heart, which is the seat of your compassion for fallible others.

Remember that *the boat is empty!*

Control your own self-talk about adversities and frustrations that you encounter in your daily life.

The Buddhists and the Stoics are in agreement that anger is created by the individual who experiences it. However, in E-CENT, we emphasize that the environmental trigger is a *necessary*, though *not sufficient*, condition for the anger to arise. (And people are *socialized creatures of habit*, and <u>not</u> individuals who go around 'making their minds up' how to think-feel about things!)

Where we agree with the Buddhists and the Stoics is in saying: If anybody to going to reduce your anger, then that must be YOU. Of all the variables in creating your anger, YOU are the only bit over which you have some control. You normally cannot control the environmental trigger (the pushy person who jumps in front of you on the queue [or line]; the car that cuts you up on the motorway [highway, autobahn]), so you will perforce be obliged to focus on controlling your own contribution to your anger. (Accept the things you cannot change and change the things you can [like your sleep sufficiency, diet, exercise, stress level, and philosophy of life).

Shrink your 'hungry ghost' ego-state by meditating on the 'emptiness' of life, and the transitory nature of your own existence. Because our ego-image is normally false - a self- and social-construct - we are in fact like ghosts, wandering around hungrily looking for experiences to feed this 'ghost' – to make it feel substantial – to make it feel good about itself. This is the "hungry ghost" image created by Buddhists to help us to realize that we are not what we seem. And it is this "hungry ghost" that bumps into others in ways that induce it to anger itself at other people and the world.

Teach yourself that you are OK exactly the way you are, and that you do not need to defeat others in order to be OK. The reason anger is so seductive is that it helps to 'concretize' our hungry ghost status; to make us feel 'holier than thou'; to encourage the belief that 'I'm OK, and you're not-OK'!

To counteract these tendencies, Buddhism encourages its adherents to adopt the precept: "I will not harm others". And harm can be done to others by shouting at them; scowling at them; speaking in a sarcastic or scathing manner with them; putting them down.

To avoid harming others, Buddhism teaches us to identify with them. As Schopenhauer says: "We are all *fellow sufferers!*" We are all part of the same reality; we are all in the same boat[93]; and we should express loving kindness towards others, as they should express loving kindness towards us.

We should practice patience with others, as they should practice patience with us.

We should meditate in order to calm our minds, to minimize stress and overreactions. We should practice mindfulness, being aware of our thoughts and feelings as they come and go.

We should not *identify with* our feelings, but just let them rise and fall within us.

We must never act out our angry thoughts or feelings. If necessary, sit in meditation, with your angry feelings swirling in your mind. Focus on them; do not try to push them away; do not try to justify them; do not feed them; just watch them. Try to experience compassion for both yourself and the other actors in your angry mind scene. Breathe deeply, and count your breaths, in and out.

Remember that it takes great courage not to act on your anger; and it is a sign of great weakness when you act out your anger. The great forcefulness of your anger, if you express it, or act on it, is a precise measure of your weakness as a truly human person. Expressing anger feeds it; focusing awareness on anger shrinks it. (Awareness. Awareness. Awareness).

Replace your anger with non-anger. Learn to communicate assertively, reasonably, respectfully:

Say: "I'm sorry, but I happen to be angry with you"[94]. There is no need to shout, or act out. Just share what is true. (Or, as taught by Claude Steiner, the TA theorist and practitioner, just say: "When you [do X], I feel [Y]...")[95].

Say: "I did not like it when you (did X). I feel angry about that. I am sorry". If necessary, ask for the change of behaviour that you consider to be justified. (The system that Helen Hall Clinard teaches is this: Say, "When you [did P], I felt [Q], because of [R, which is a tangible effect upon me or my personal domain]; and I would like you to do [S] instead")[96].

Feeling anger is not something to celebrate. Feeling anger does not entitle you to a medal of self-justification, or self-righteousness; or a certificate confirming that "You were right; and they were wrong!"

~~~

Additional Antidotes

Here are some additional antidotes that should help[97]. Write out the two or three that help you the most, and carry them with you.

The Law of Karma says that we reap what we sow. Therefore, we must have done something to have earned this frustration with which we are now faced. If we respond angrily, we will worsen our karma. If we learn to roll with the blows, we may be able to improve our future karma. (The law of karma is the law of cause and effect).

Accept the things you cannot change, and change the things you can. This principle also occurs in Stoicism.

Realistic analysis – If somebody says something bad about me, is there some bit with which I can agree? 'Nobody is perfect'.

Realization of 'emptiness': If you understand that we live in a sea of language, and we are always dealing with linguistic categories as if they were 'concrete realities' – and we are always interpreting everything, and not seeing it 'as it is' - you might experience the 'emptiness of everything'.

Openness: Be willing to listen to the complaints of others, and to talk them through. Perhaps the problem can be solved to your mutual satisfaction. Do you really need to go to war over their current perception of the problem?

Relativity: Is this problem really worth fretting about, and getting worked up about? On a scale of one to ten, how bad is it? If I knew I was going to die next week, how significant would this problem seem today?

Change your methods of motivation: Are you getting angry with others to persuade them to follow your lead? If so, it would be better for everybody if you changed your methods, and learned the skills of persuasion, instead of coercion. If your ideas are as valuable and correct as you currently think, it should not be too difficult to figure out how to sell your ideas to others, instead of browbeating them.

Don't make fists and angry faces: If you clench your fists and scowl when you are engaged in an encounter with somebody, you will feel tense and angry; and they will see you as tense and angry, and they may respond in kind (because they can pick up your angry state via their 'mirror neurons' – even if you are trying to hide your nonverbal signals)[98]. Practice physical relaxation, and try to calm yourself at the beginning, during the middle, and at the end of each day.

~~~

Get your anger under reasonable control

Chapter 11. The General CBT Position on Anger

Background

CBT began its 'official' life as Cognitive Therapy (CT), created by Dr Aaron Tim Beck, about ten years *after* Dr Ellis published his first book on Rational therapy (REBT) [99], which is seen by many as the ('unofficial') *original form* of cognitive behavioural therapy.

Eventually Beckian CT was bracketed together with REBT, and some other Cognitive and Rational therapies (including those of Meichenbaum and Maultsby) under the umbrella term Cognitive Behaviour Therapy (CBT).

The approach of Cognitive Therapy to emotional self-management began with the work of Dr Aaron Tim Beck – Beck, 1976/1989[100] - who was strongly influenced by Dr Albert Ellis.

We do not promote the theories of Dr Albert Ellis, because, although he had some good ideas, he was also not just a sceptic and a moderate Stoic; he was an Extreme Stoic; and tried to teach the world to put up with unreasonable abuse and oppression; and he implicitly blamed his clients for their own upset emotions. ("What are *you doing* to make yourself upset?" he would demand to know!)

Because Beck was a medical doctor, he set about his research in a different manner from Ellis, who was a philosopher and psychologist; and thus Beck created a different range of distinctions to explain human emotional disturbance. (In a later book, Beck did adopt a more philosophical approach)[101]. Beck has his own limitations, but we will review his work on anger here, to see what we can mine from it.

Beck on anger

Beck links his understanding of anger back to the way in which a primitive organism will try to destroy or repel a noxious agent that tries to invade it. From this he infers a basic pattern in humans to respond angrily when they are physically or verbally attacked. However, Beck recognizes that this does not always apply, and he cited Ellis (1962) in support of the conclusion that people do not respond angrily to offence if they see the offending agent as being "justified, non-arbitrary or reasonable". (Beck, 1976/89, page 65).

It is also important to note, here, that people do not respond angrily to offence if they are *afraid of the consequences!*

The common thread that Beck thinks runs through most instances of anger arousal is this: "The main character (or protagonist) is subjected to an unpleasant experience (the offence) by one or more adversaries. He is the object of deliberate physical attack, criticism, coercion, thwarting, rejection, deprivation, or opposition. These situations are noxious because they encroach on the protagonist's safety, self-esteem, or desires; they are perceived as a deliberate, direct impingement on his domain. Even when the offence is not motivated by malice, it may be perceived as such by the protagonist". (Page 66).

Beck also recognizes that an individual may feel angry in response to commands and restrictions which seem to him to be encroaching on his rights. These rights may include: "autonomy, freedom of action, and freedom of expression, (and) also expectations of respect, courtesy, consideration, and loyalty from other people".

Transgressions against an individual's expectations and personal rules may arise in situations of various types: "(1) direct and intentional attack; (2) direct, unintentional attack; (3) violation of laws, standards, social mores; hypothetical threats, sub-standard behaviour, breach of idiosyncratic moral code." (Page 71).

According to Beck: "The common factor for arousal of anger is the individual's appraisal of an assault on his domain, including his values, moral code, and protective rules. This factor, while a necessary condition, is not sufficient in itself to arouse anger. In order to provoke anger, other specific conditions must be present. First, the individual must take the infringement seriously and label it negatively. ... Second, the individual must not consider the noxious situation an immediate or continuing danger. If he is concerned primarily with his own safety, he will be more anxious than angry. Third, the individual must focus primarily on the wrongfulness of the offense and the offender rather than on any injury he may have sustained". (Pages 71-72)

Evaluation

That is a very helpful consideration of the 'A's (or Activating offences) and the 'B's (or Beliefs-appraisals and thought-conclusions) of an individual in an anger-inducing situation.

By contrast with Beck, Dr Albert Ellis's REBT explains the 'internal component' of emotional disturbances, including anger, as a result of a person holding *irrational beliefs* consisting of 'demands'; and 'awfulizings' and 'damning their adversary'. This approach has influenced many CBT therapists, who have adopted Ellis's ABC model as follows:

A: Activating event: Something happens of an insulting or frustrating nature (such as a friend or colleague walking past you as you are about to greet them, as if they are discounting you.

B: Belief system: You believe you are being slighted, which my must not be, and that this is as bad as can be.

C: Emotional consequence: Anger.

Ellis discounted everything except your Beliefs in causing anger. He believed that nobody needs to anger themselves about anything, which is the Extreme Stoic view – based on the idea that "nobody can harm you".

Some modern CBTers, even some who have been influenced by Ellis, but also by psychological training, include more than your belief; such as the contribution of the automatic physiological stress response; being tired; but mostly they focus upon self-talk; beliefs; distorted evaluations; etc. (see Dr Ann Macaskill's 2002 book).

~~~

Dr Aaron Tim Beck's CT attributes all emotional disturbances to the presence of 'negative automatic thoughts' (NATs), or distorted thinking processes.

According to Beck, a person has a noxious experience (at point 'A' in the ABC model). Then (at point 'B'), s/he surfaces an *automatic thought*, which s/he may or may not notice. And that automatic thought causes his/her anger.

But what are these kinds of automatic thoughts? They have now been refined into a fairly standard list, as for example in Dr David Burns' book on Cognitive Therapy (CT).[102]

David Burns on NATs

The most common automatic thoughts in CT/CBT are as follows (as presented in my own words – because most of the CBT labels sound so similar to each other, and give the appearance of excessive overlapping of concepts. My wording is intended to clarify these distinctions to make the differences between them more apparent to the reader):

1. <u>Black and white thinking</u>: Everything is seen as totally good or totally bad. There are no shades of grey.

2. <u>Always and never thinking</u>: The person believes that 'it' – some noxious experience – life, or some part of it – will always be this way and never get better.

3. <u>Tunnel vision</u>: The person tends to focus on one event/ object/ problem to the exclusion of all other events/ objects.

4. <u>Jumping to conclusions</u>: Based on too thin a slice of evidence, the person reaches a negative conclusion which cannot be justified. This can include Negative Mind Reading, and Negative Fortune Telling.

5. <u>Emotional reasoning</u>: The person uses their feelings as 'evidence' that something is wrong. "I would not be feeling so upset if there was not some good reason for it".

6. <u>Demandingness</u>: This is the inappropriate use of absolute *shoulds* and *musts* to describe our preferences.

7. <u>Labelling</u>: This means that one extrapolates from a bad behaviour or poor performance, by another person, to a 'global negative rating' of that other person as a whole, who is then labelled: 'evil', 'bar-steward', 'loser', 'fool', 'failure', 'son of a b----', and so on.

8. <u>Self-blaming and self-damning</u>: A person may damn themselves as a whole being when they get negative feedback from the world. "I am a louse for acting badly".

Burns (1990) does not distinguish between anger on the one hand, and irritation and annoyance on the other, which REBT theorists do. Neither does he write of the distinction between 'healthy' and 'unhealthy' anger.

CBT uses its own version of the ABC model, in which something noxious happens at point 'A', which is the 'Activating event'. Then the individual to whom it happens has some automatic thoughts about the 'A', at point 'B' in the model, which is their Belief system. And finally, at point 'C', anger is caused by those automatic thoughts about the noxious activating event.

According to Burns (1990), page 16, the most common automatic thoughts that result in anger are as follows:

- **Should statements**: For example: *He should not have said that nasty thing to me.* Or: *She's got no right to treat me that way.*

- **Labelling**: *He's a son-of-a-b----*

- **Mind reading**: "She obviously doesn't have any respect for me".

- **Blaming**: "This is entirely his fault".

- **All-or-nothing thinking**: "I'm right and she's wrong about this".

- **Overgeneralization**: "All she ever thinks about is herself".

It is not too difficult to imagine a person uttering one of these statements, to themselves, and then feeling angry. However, it is not at all clear that the statement came before the feeling. The feeling could well be an automatic, habit-based Response (R) to a Stimulus (S), based on the total state of the Organism (O): including diet, exercise, self-talk, sleep, relaxation experiences, stress level, and so on.

From a E-CENT perspective, these examples of disturbed thinking are most likely linked into networks of thinking-feeling-acting 'inferences' – called 'frames' – which may also include some of the key REBT inferences and irrational beliefs. When one of the inferences in a frame is triggered (non-consciously) they are all triggered (non-consciously) and the linked emotion is then fired up. Thus, in E-CENT, the anger is not caused by one of the statements above, but rather by the whole network of linked cognitive-emotive inferences, and bodily responses, which are all linked together to a habitual emotional response.

CBT strategies

Common CBT strategies for curbing anger are summarized by Dr Sarah Edelman (2006)[103] as follows:

"A number of cognitive strategies can help to release anger, including

- A cost-benefit analysis,

- Goal-directed thinking,

- Thought monitoring and disputation,

- Empathy, and

- Coping statements.

"Accepting that injustice is unavoidable at times, and that justice is sometimes subjective, can also help to release anger.

"Behavioural strategies that are helpful in the management of anger include

- Problem solving, and:

- Arousal reduction techniques such as physical exercise and deep relaxation[104].

"In addition

- Behavioural disputing – choosing to behave in a friendly manner towards someone we resent can be a powerful strategy for releasing anger.

- Utilizing effective communication can also resolve anger by reducing interpersonal tensions". (Page 114).

~~~

Chapter 12: The E-CENT theory of anger

Introduction

Emotive-Cognitive Embodied Narrative Therapy (E-CENT) is a relatively new system of counselling and therapy which grew out of my enquiries into the core models of Rational Therapy (REBT).

The basic perspective of E-CENT theory is this:

Emotion is primary, because it is innate. Cognition is secondary, and always linked to, and supported by, emotion.

And emotive-cognitive functioning is shaped by the socialization process of mother and child interaction. The mind is a socialized function of the body-brain, and is mainly wired up in the form of social experiences, which are often understood in the form of socialized stories or narratives; though many experiences probably remain un-narrativized: (visual or kinesthetic records of 'something' that happened).

E-CENT theory evolved at a time when I was exploring the foundations of REBT theory, plus aspects of Transactional Analysis (TA), moral philosophy, elements of Zen Buddhism, Object Relations theory and Attachment theory. (Overall, I have studied thirteen different systems of counselling and therapy – formally, at post-master's level – plus four or five more since completing my doctorate in counselling).

E-CENT, as it emerged, originally had many marks of REBT and its other contributing systems upon it; but it has evolved to become increasingly different from REBT and most of those other systems in several significant respects.

E-CENT theory of aggression

The E-CENT perspective on aggression and anger is, as suggested elsewhere in this book, an integration of:

(1) The theory of innate aggression described by Lorenz (1966/2002), and:

(2) The social learning theory of aggression developed by Bandura et al (1961)[105]. Plus:

(3) An understanding of how particular states of the body, induced by adequate or inadequate diet, exercise and sleep, can create tendencies towards angry outbursts, or to reduce our capacity to manage our angry urges.

Figure 12.1 below shows three elements:

(1) the innate aggression of the *id* (which is German for the 'it' - or *the physical child* as it was at birth – an 'object' more than a subject, but with the developmental potential to become a 'person');

(2) the socially shaped and innate aggression of the *super-ego* (which is internalized memories of mother); and:

(3) the compromise approach to aggression of the **ego**/self:

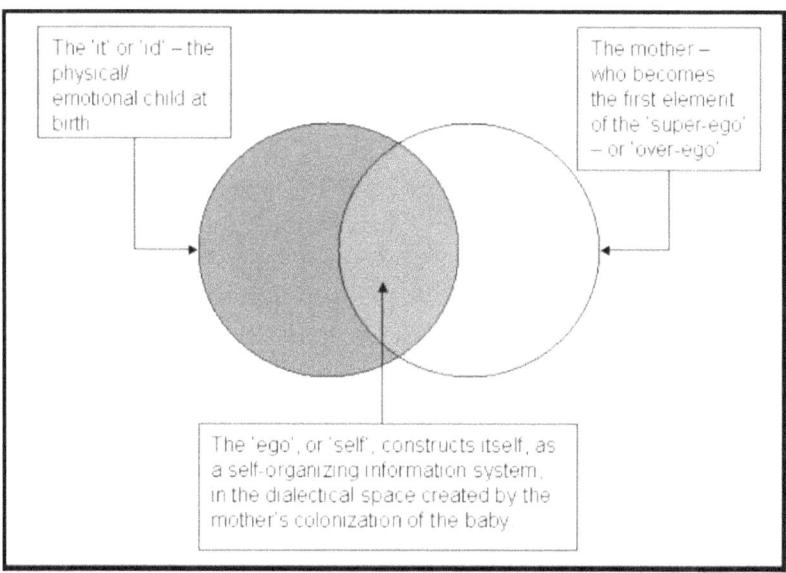

Figure 12.1: The most basic model of E-CENT – The interactive (or dialectical) nature of the individual/social ego.

The first thing to note about Figure 12.1 is this:

The ego (which begins as overlapping [or interweaving] of mother and child) is a product of relationship, and cannot exist without (external and/or internalized) relationship.

Secondly, because each baby is unique, with its own unique genetic heritage, and because every mother is unique, the ego will also be unique – including having a unique pattern of *aggressive arousal* and *anger activation* threshold.

This means that we will each have a somewhat different degree of aggression (innately) and a significantly different degree of aggression-restraint and aggression-modelling, depending upon who our mothers and fathers and school teachers happened to be, and the kind of general social environment in which we grew up. (We have already seen above how anger is linked to attachment patterns, and now we can see how this occurs).

Next we must consider the E-CENT theory of the good/bad innate split – the inheritance of a Good and Bad Wolf state in every human.

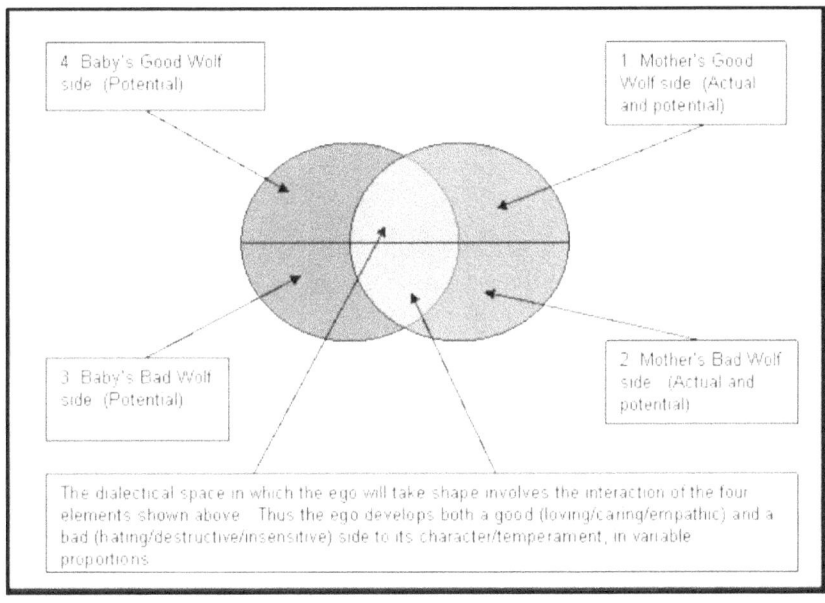

Figure 12.2 – The good and bad sides of human nature/culture

The good and bad wolf are inherent in human nature, and in human culture, and the proportions are variable in each individual over time, and from situation to situation

Figure 12.2 shows our understanding of the split nature of all humans, between a good side and an evil side – commonly referred to in E-CENT as the *Good Wolf* and the *Bad Wolf*. However, unlike in the case of Freud's

Thanatos and *Eros* urges, we do not see aggression as *belonging* exclusively to the Bad Wolf.

Aggression can occur from either state: e.g. healthy anger from the Good Wolf and unhealthy anger from the Bad Wolf.

In E-CENT we see **healthy anger** as *constructive aggression* – normally assertion of legitimate and reasonable rights of the individual – which stops us being exploited or abused – and which prevents us going too far in attacking others for our own benefit.

We see **unhealthy anger** as excessive or inappropriate use of aggression against others (or the self) in pursuit of some unjustified goals, including unreasonable or unrealistic demands, or in the acting out of a dysfunctional relationship history: (See Appendix D, below).

Unhealthy anger may also arise because our basic needs are not being met, including problems of social isolation, inadequate diet or sleep, insufficient physical exercise, stressful living space, abusive relationships, and so on.

What then is the E-CENT approach to managing anger, or helping others to manage their anger?

Let us begin by looking at the core model used in E-CENT, in Figure 12.3 below.

Whereas REBT and CBT begin with **the ABC model**, E-CENT counselling begins with **the Holistic SOR model**:

Figure 12.3 below shows how we present the holistic SOR model for our clients.

As indicated in Figure 12.3, E-CENT theory takes a holistic view of the client as a social-body-mind, with a habit-based character and temperament, living in a particular social and physical environment, with stressors and supports.

The client has a personal history which is unique to them; plus extensive social shaping that comes from their family of origin; and some from their community; some from their nation/ race/ gender, etc.

The Holistic Stimulus-Organism-Response Model (H-SOR)		
Column 1	Column 2	Column 3
S = Stimulus	O = Organism	R = Response
When something significant happens, which is apprehended by the organism's (or person's) nervous system, the organism is activated or aroused (positively or negatively)	The organism responds, well or badly. The incoming stimulus may activate or interact with: (1) Innate needs and tendencies; (2) Family history and attachment style; (3) Recent personal history; (4) Emotive-cognitive schemas (as guides to action); (5) Narratives, stories, frames and other storied elements (which may be hyper-activating, hypo-activating, or affect regulating); (6) Character and temperament; (7) Need satisfaction; goals and values; (8) Diet and supplementation, medication, exercise regime, sleep and relaxation histories; (9) Ongoing environmental stressors, state of current relationship(s), and satisfaction with life stages, etc., etc.	The organism outputs a response, in the form of visible behaviour and inferable emotional reactions, like anger, anxiety, depression, embarrassment, etc.

Figure 12.3: The E-CENT holistic SOR model

This illustration should be read as follows:

- Column 1 - 'S' = (equals) a **stimulus**,

- which, when experienced by an O = **Organism** (in our case a human), may activate or interact with any of the factors listed in column 2;

- and this will produce an R = **Response**, as shown in column 3.

In our present case, we can say that an angry response by a person is generated by the interaction of all of the factors listed in column 2 of the Holistic-SOR model, though some elements from column 2 may have more influence than others at particular times.

To be more precise: The holistic SOR model states that a client (a person) responds (angrily or non-angrily) at point 'R', to a (negative or positive) stimulus at point 'S', on the basis of the current state of their social-body-mind.

How well rested are they? How many hours sleep do they get each night?

How high or low is their blood-sugar level (which is related to diet and nutrition)?

Do they eat junk foods containing trans-fats (which have been shown to cause anger outbursts)?

Do they eat enough omega-3 fatty acids (which are highly concentrated in oily fish, like salmon, sardine, mackerel, etc.; which have been shown to lower levels of aggression among violent criminals in prison experiments)?

How well connected are they to significant others (which is a measure of social support)?

How much conflict do they have at home or at work?

How much angry modelling did they see in the behaviour of their parents when they were very young? And/or in their school peers; school teachers; etc. And in violent movies at an impressionable age? (Remember the Bobo doll experiments on learned aggressiveness).

What other pressures are bearing down upon them (e.g. from their socio-economic circumstances; physical health; home/ housing; work/ income; security/ insecurity; etc.)

And how emotionally intelligent are they? (Emotional intelligence is, of course, learned, and can be re-learned!)

Within the Holistic-SOR model (in Figure 12.3 above), in the middle column, what we are aiming to do is to construct a balance sheet (in our heads) of the **pressures** bearing down on the client (person), and the **coping resources** that they have for dealing with those pressures.

~~~

So this is a **historical-social-stress model**. It is not a purely 'cognitive distortion' model; nor a purely 'biological/sexual urges' model; nor a purely 'prizing and listening' model.

~~~

Sometimes working on a person's *philosophy of life* – or 'self-talk' or 'inner dialogue' - will help them to reduce or control their anger; but they also have to work on their body, via physical fitness, adequate nutrition, sufficient good-quality sleep, and various other factors. For example, eating junk foods, high in trans-facts, has been shown to cause individuals to develop anger management problems. By contrast, introducing young, violent prisoners to a diet high in omega-3 fats, has been found to reduce incidents of violence or aggressive conflict dramatically.

And they may also have to go back and dig up some aspects of their past history, and to *complete* (or *digest*) stressful or traumatic experiences that were left undigested at some time in their (early) past. (See Appendix D).

~~~

But, as indicated above, *philosophy of life* is also important. Here is an example of me working on my philosophy of life, or reframing an experience, related to anger:

> Let us imagine I am attending a social event, say a party, and I am engaged in a conversation with several individuals around a table. Unexpectedly, one of them *implies* that I do not deserve to earn very much money, unlike certain bank officials; and that I am probably worth about the same amount of money that a pensioner gets.
>
> Suddenly I feel very angry towards this person. What has happened?
>
> **E = Event =** Somebody has insulted me, and impugned my value to society, and my earning potential, and thus my social status…
>
> **F = Frame or Framing =** I automatically, and non-consciously, 'view' this statement through a particular lens, or 'frame of reference' (which is both physical and psychological, based in my body-brain-mind), and which is unknowable to me …
>
> **R = Response =** I unaccountably, and quite against my conscious wishes, feel a strong desire to hit the person who insulted me, or to at least call him some ugly name. But I (manage to) restrain myself, (perhaps) because I have never been good at physical or verbal battles (and am therefore not in the habit of responding aggressively to insults); and I (may) also (be wired up by my experience to) consider it 'unseemly' to respond aggressively to others in company. For some minutes I continue to be unable to think

straight. I feel unhappy. My guts and emotive-cogitations are churning (throughout my body-brain-mind). Gradually I regain my composure (because my orbitofrontal cortex [OFC] has regained control of my limbic system – automatically]. But my feelings towards the individual who has insulted me have now switched from being *too hot* to being *decidedly cool* and *distant*.

How did I get control of my anger? Firstly, I (might, non-consciously have) reminded myself of this statement by Marcus Aurelius (which I have read many times!):

"Say to yourself in the early morning: I shall meet today inquisitive, ungrateful, violent, treacherous, envious, uncharitable men (and women). All these things have come upon them through ignorance of real good and ill…" (Aurelius, 1991, page 7)[106].

If I did this, then it would have occurred automatically, because I have trained myself to have this belief, hard-wired into my non-conscious mind.

And secondly, I (may have) reminded myself of the Buddha's insight (which is expressed in my Window No.1, above), that all humans suffer frustrations and difficulties much of the time. *So why must I – a 'special doll' – be exempt from suffering?* (And perhaps) no good reason could be found.

Again, if I did this, then I did it automatically, because I have trained myself over time to believe what the Buddha taught. (I cannot summon up *conscious philosophical solutions* by choice on the spur of the moment! I am *a creature of habit*, and unless I learned to have a particular philosophy of life, by sheer effort of determined learning, in the past, then I could not expect a statement from the Buddha to pop into my mind in this context!)

~~~

So let us now take a look at some of the key points about anger that underpin the E-CENT approach.

Firstly, Anger is innate…

Anger is part of our innate 'fight or flight response', which helped to keep us alive through millions of years of evolution. We need to know when to fight, when to retreat, when to eat, and when to reproduce: there are the five F's: fight, flee, freeze, feed and fornicate.

In very young babies we can see evidence of innate anger at frustration, and as children reach the age of two years, this can become very pronounced.

Secondly, Anger is socially shaped...

From the beginning of life, the new child is in almost constant interaction with its mother, or main carer, who works relentlessly to shape the child's behavior. *Do this; do not do that; this is okay; that is not okay.* This social shaping includes *modelling* or *promoting* particular approaches to 'legitimate anger' and penalizing or scolding the child for 'inappropriate anger'. (In some families, *all anger is outlawed*; and in some families, anger is *the main emotion that is allowed*, and tenderness is outlawed!)

If you had the good fortune to be borne into a family in which you could establish a secure attachment to your mother/carer, and your mother and father had good control over their own anger expression, then you are unlikely to have many problems with your own anger today.

However, if you had angry parents, or even one angry parent and one passive parent, and you failed to establish a secure attachment to your mother and father, then you are likely to have some problems with managing your anger today.

(However, you can still learn how to control your anger today, despite your childhood experiences, if you find the right kind of counsellor/ therapist; or you study the right kind of anger management literature).

~~~

Third, Anger is linked to the body and mind...

In Emotive-Cognitive Embodied Narrative Therapy (E-CENT), we have integrated the somatic, neurobiological and cognitive theories of anger causation – plus attachment theory, and affect regulation theory, etc. - into a new, more complex model, which seems to us to fit the facts better than any preceding model on its own.

This model shows why it is not enough to ask an angry person "What are you *telling yourself* about (X) in order to make yourself angry?"

This is so because the person's anger level is partly driven by

- their emotional sensitivity (which is genetically determined);

- partly by the culture and sub-culture(s) from which they come (because of social learning);

- and partly from their physiological state resulting from their use, or lack of use, of physical exercise, healthy diet, stimulants, relaxation techniques, etc.

Thus E-CENT theory takes into account the various potential sources of anger of the individual, while REBT mainly focuses on their self-talk. Back in 2003-2009, when I began to experiment with modifying/updating the ABC model, to move it from a simple model to a complex model, I added back the body, which changed the whole theory of human emotional disturbance.

This is explored in the following illustration.

Earlier, we looked at the E-CENT model of brain-mind-body-environment connection and interaction, as follows:

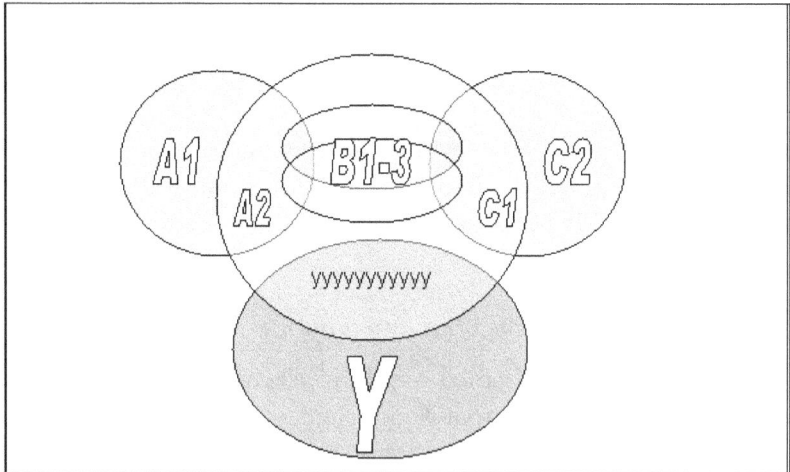

Figure 12.4 - The A>B>Y>y>C Model al la Humphrey-Byrne Linkages

Figure 12.4 shows the human body, represented by the darker grey ellipse (big Y); and the head/brain/mind as the large circle in the middle of the frame.

Using the model in Figure 12.4, we would say that a stimulus at A1 (outside the person) triggers an interpretive inference at A2, which triggers an evaluative (cognitive-emotive) processing of that signal at B1-3. The B1 or 2 or 3 (described in detail in Byrne 2009c)[107], then sends out *at least* three signals. One goes to the face-body to initiate a physiological response. One goes to the collection of little internal y's, (inside the B boundary – in the brain/mind/body) representing *the personal history of physiological responses to previous stimuli* of the type apprehended at A2. And one goes straight to the C1 to signal an affective (or emotive/behavioural) output. The brain-based little y's yield up the best fit to Stimulus A2 of *historically appropriate* physiological arousal, and send a signal to C1 containing that information. (This is similar to what is called 'pattern matching' in the 'Human Givens' tradition: Griffin and Tyrrell, 2004[108] [See Chapter 13, below]).

We could say a lot more about the relationships between the various elements of the body-mind in Figure 12.4, but the main point is clear. Human emotion is based in the body-mind, and that includes anger arousal. Anger is not caused by 'irrational beliefs' or 'automatic thoughts'. That explanation is too simple, or, rather, simplistic, when considered in the context of the middle column of the Holistic-SOR model.

Fourth, Anger can be controlled by controlling your body and mind...

Because the body-mind is one integrated system, we can tackle anger (and other emotions) through our bodies and through our minds; but preferably through a combination of the two.

Recommended solutions to problems of anger in E-CENT include:

1. Learning to be assertive, instead of aggressive. (See Appendix C).

2. Learning to give up being a Blamer, and become a Leveller. See Appendix B).

3. Reviewing and changing diet, exercise, sleep and self-talk approaches. (See Appendix A, below).

4. Reframing the anger-inducing stimulus/event. For example, by using the Six Windows model, described in Chapter 3, above.

5. Giving up unreasonable and/or unrealistic demands, desires or expectations of life.

6. Recognizing that humans are creatures of habit, and products of imperfect socialization processes. They are like 'boats emerging from the fog, with no pilot (or, at best, a sleeping pilot)!'

7. Learning to forgive those individuals who transgress against us and our needs, desires, wants and moral rules (on the understanding that our time will come when we need the forgiveness of others!). See Chapter 2, above.

8. Giving up exaggerating the degree of badness of the anger-inducing stimulus/event. ("Life could always be worse than this!")

9. Giving up blaming and judging myself, other people and the world, and substituting the 'I'm OK – You're OK' position, as described in the section on Transactional Analysis.

10. Compassion or radical acceptance: Learning to accept yourself and other people *on one condition* (and that one condition is that you, and they, must commit to acting morally). This is explored briefly in Byrne, (2010b)[109].

~~~

Chapter 13: The 'Human Givens' approach to anger

Introduction

The 'Human Givens' approach to emotions in general, and anger in particular, was developed by Joe Griffin and Ivan Tyrrell, two psychologists who wanted to integrate what is known about human needs with psychological theory to produce an integrative system of counselling and therapy.

In their 2004 book, they argued that

> "…anger is mostly not an appropriate reaction for normal minor irritations; the smooth running of social intercourse is more often better served when it is inhibited. But there are times when anger could be vital to our survival, to defend ourselves from physical attack, and we need access to it. Fortunately, the (outer brain) cortex is infinitely malleable and we can do that. It is a wonderfully flexible system whereby the instinctive core personality is kept intact but its expression can continually readapt to different circumstances". (Page 43, Griffin and Tyrrell, 2004).

Their argument is that dreaming has a lot to do with keeping the core instincts intact, despite our daytime adaptations to a controlling or regulating culture.

Their argument can be readily understood in the context of a consideration of the overlapping circles model of E-CENT.

Human Givens and the E-CENT theory

In E-CENT theory we see the new-born baby being colonized by the mother, so that an overlapping psychic space emerges, in the objective, social world, which is also internalized in the mind of both mother and baby.

This is how we normally depict that state (items 1 and 2 below; but item 3 has been added to show how the Human Givens theory fits into our model):

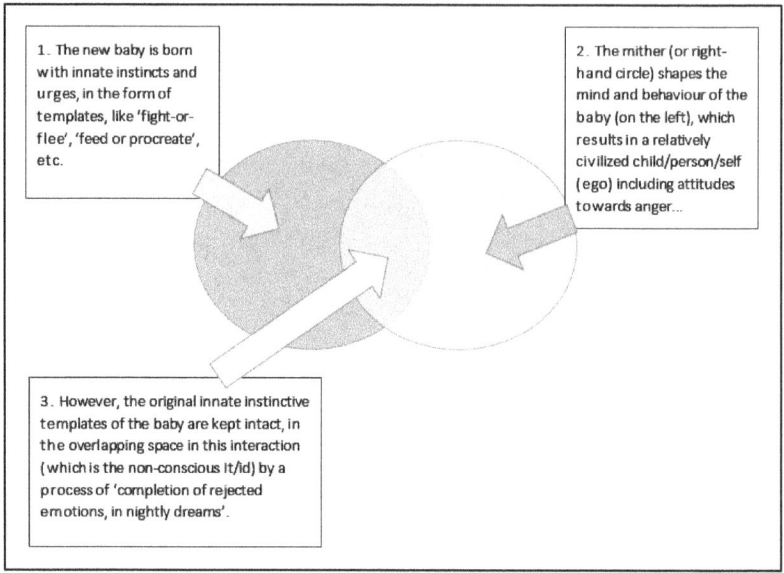

1. The new baby is born with innate instincts and urges, in the form of templates, like 'fight-or-flee', 'feed or procreate', etc.

2. The mither (or right-hand circle) shapes the mind and behaviour of the baby (on the left), which results in a relatively civilized child/person/self (ego) including attitudes towards anger...

3. However, the original innate instinctive templates of the baby are kept intact, in the overlapping space in this interaction (which is the non-conscious It/id) by a process of 'completion of rejected emotions, in nightly dreams'.

Figure 13.1: Integrating the HG theory and the E-CENT theory

In our waking states, we (human individuals) are guided by our socialized ego – which is the middle/overlapping space in the illustration above – which was shaped by the interactions and tensions of

- our instinctive body-mind (or 'id', or 'it' – the left-hand circle) with

- mother and father (or superego – the right-hand circle).

But when we sleep, we get to 'complete' any 'id arousal' that was blocked by the socialized ego. This keeps our innate instinctive 'templates' (such as the fight-or-flight response) intact, despite our socialization. (Compare with Griffin and Tyrrell, 2004, pages 41-44).

These authors also see patterns of anger response to current frustrations as forms of 'post hypnotic suggestion' – rather than behavioural reinforcement – which comes from the 'trances' induced in us as children in our families, in which our parents implicitly said: "This is how to deal with frustration", etc.

Thus, they suggest, "...when carrying out a posthypnotic suggestion, we are, effectively, in the dream state". (Page 70). Or, using my model above, we can say, we are operating from pure 'non-socialized id', and not our socialized ego.

This seems a little muddled to me. If I am acting out of a trance state induced by my parents during my socialization, then I am acting from my (non-consciously) socialized ego, and not from my (pure, unreformed) id/it!

~~~

The complete HG theory of anger

In 2008, Griffin and Tyrrell published a book on the subject of controlling anger, which elaborates the Human Givens (HG) theory. Their core argument is that the function of anger is to help us to defend ourselves and our territory. Anger is part of the fight-or-flight response, which is managed automatically from the amygdala, which is part of the 'emotional brain'. Activation of the amygdala disrupts our 'thinking brain' (centred in the neocortex, and especially the frontal lobes) and puts emotion in control of our functioning. (But, in E-CENT theory, we argue that we are always controlled and directed by socialized emotional experience. Or socialized perceiving-feeling-thinking-acting!)

According to the basic HG theory, we are pattern-matching organisms. We store patterns of experience, and when we have new experiences, we (automatically, non-consciously) match them to previous patterns, in order to know how to deal with them. (This fits very well with the E-CENT theory).

This seems to me to be a form of schema theory, from constructivism, e.g. Piaget and Gibson. The basic implication is this: When we meet a noxious (insulting, frustrating) stimulus, we may match it to one from the past - which we responded to with an angry response - and that is then how we respond when we encounter a very similar noxious stimulus in the here and now. Those patterns are linked to the amygdala, in the limbic system, which they also call the 'emotional brain'. But in E-CENT theory we would say, those patterns are not just linked to the amygdala, but also to the orbitofrontal cortex (OFC), the role of which is to try to damp down excessive arousal from the emotional brain. (But the 'wiring' of the OFC is a result of socialized experiences, so, we may have a tendency to crank our emotions upwards [into anger or anxiety], downwards [into depression, shame, etc.], or to keep them on an even keel [calm, un-rattled, etc.] –

depending on *what we learned* from our family of origin, our schooling, and so on).

When we match a pattern that triggers anger in us, adrenaline is pumped into our bloodstream; we automatically breathe faster to get more oxygen; our blood pressure goes up; blood is diverted away from digestion to limb animation; glucose is freed up to provide energy for action; and our bodies are flooded with the stress hormone, cortisol.

People may be more prone to having angry outbursts if they do not get enough sleep; are physically unwell; when their blood sugar level is dropped by hunger; when they are experiencing withdrawal from something addictive; during hormonal swings in women; or when we are in chronic or acute pain.

When *the fight response* is triggered in a person, they can only 'think emotionally', in black and white terms. This results in jumping to (often wrong) conclusions; blaming people; sweeping generalizations; taking up rigid, prejudicial positions; and exaggerated, extreme reactions which are over the top.

Anger, in the Human Givens theory, is not just about our evaluations and beliefs, but also includes the component that "something is not working in (the) lives" of people who are angry. In the terms of the ABC model, this means that people are not just upset by their beliefs (at point B), but ALSO, and perhaps more so, by *their need deprivations* (at A). "Every one of us is born with innate needs that must be met..." (Page 39). The concept of the "human givens" is about our innate needs and the responses we have been given by nature to meet them.

Human Needs

According to the HG approach, we have physical needs – like warmth, shelter, sleep, food and drink. And we have emotional needs, which include:

- Security – the need to feel safe;
- A sense of autonomy and control over our lives;
- Receiving and giving attention;
- Friendship, love, intimacy;

- The sense of belonging to a group;

- Personal space and privacy;

- A sense of status;

- A sense of competence and achievement;

- A sense of meaning and purpose.

~~~

Innate Human Responses

Our abilities and action tendencies which help us to get our needs met include the following:

- The ability to learn and remember; to add new knowledge to 'innate knowledge'.

- The ability to empathize and connect with other humans;

- Our emotions and instincts;

- Our problem-solving imagination;

- Our ability to think, plan, analyze and adapt;

- Our ability to understand the world unconsciously – through 'pattern matching';

- The ability to be 'more objective' – to 'observe ourselves relatively objectively'. (?);

- The ability to discharge unexperienced (or repressed) emotions during our dream sleep.

~~~

Barriers to need satisfaction

According to Griffin and Tyrrell (2008), three things can go wrong which can stop us getting our needs met:

1. If our social environment is unhealthy, and we grow up with emotional dysfunctions, such as unhealthy anger; and/or:

2. The brain-mind may be damaged by genetic damage or trauma. Traumatized individuals may be constantly stressed, and likely to misidentify 'patterns' that call up anger inappropriately; and/or:

3. The innate guidance system is not being used properly. For example, parents may encourage their children to develop learned helplessness; or some other dysfunctional belief/behaviour system. We may learn to be non-confident at home or in school. We might over-use our imagination to keep replaying bad memories, which constantly upset us.

~~~

Reasons for excessive anger

Here are some reasons, given by Griffin and Tyrrell (2008) for excessive anger:

• A build-up of stress. (Too many demands on your coping resources).

• Lack of negotiation skills. (If we don't ask for what we want we may be put upon and not get our needs met. We may do this for a while, and then explode).

• Low self-esteem can make us sensitive to 'perceived slights'. Low self-esteem may drive sexual jealousy, leading to violent outbursts in relationships.

• Antisocial individuals have difficulty relating to others, which can be frustrating, which in turn can trigger anger.

• Some people may be addicted to the adrenaline rush caused by engaging in angry outbursts.

• People may react angrily when they are actually fearful. They may lash out at (what they perceived to be) a frightening threat.

• People may get angry in the present because of some unexpressed anger about humiliation in the past. (Pages 66-75).

• Sometimes women become angry with their partners because their partner is too cerebral or not empathic enough.

• Sometimes men become angry at their partner because their partner is 'too illogical' or not systematic enough.

~~~

The HG approach to reducing and controlling anger

Griffin and Tyrrell (2008) offer the following advice for overcoming anger:

1. Learn how to relax:

    a.   Relaxed breathing;

    b.   Whole body approaches.

2. Live more healthily:

    a.   Manage your diet better;

    b.   Take regular physical exercise;

    c.   Get a good night's sleep.

3. Do an 'emotional needs assessment' on yourself - (This is based on a scale of 1-7, where 1 = need not being met; and 7 = perfect need satisfaction).

> The emotional needs assessment deals with 'activating events', such as: Receiving attention from others; or Having an intimate relationship. While others seem to be 'emotional Consequences' (in the language of the ABC's of REBT): such as, Feeling connected to others; or Feeling secure. Here is the full list:
>
>   a.   Do you feel secure in all major areas of your life?
>
>   b.   Do you feel you receive enough attention?
>
>   c.   Do you think you give other people enough attention?
>
>   d.   Do you feel in control of your life most of the time?
>
>   e.   Do you feel part of the wider community?
>
>   f.   Can you obtain privacy when you need it?
>
>   g.   Do you have at least one close friend?
>
>   h.   Do you have an intimate relationship in your life?
>
>   i.   Do you feel an emotional connection to others?
>
>   j.   Do you have a status in life (whatever it may be) that you value and that is acknowledged?
>
>   k.   Are you achieving things in your life that you are proud of?

l. Do you feel competent in at least one major area of your life?

m. Are you mentally and physically stretched in ways which give you a sense of meaning and purpose?

~~~

4. Watch your 'self-talk'. (Page 116). This is based on the Human Givens systems' own ABC model, which works like this:

a. A = Awareness. (Become aware of what you are thinking. This means identifying the words you are using in your mind to describe your current situation)

b. B = Block that self-talk. When you spot an angry thought, say: "No"; or "Stop"; or "go away". Or: "No, I will not entertain that angry thought!"

c. C – Challenge your thoughts. Imagine you are a Martian, observing your angry thoughts. What do you think of them? Are they accurate? Are they helpful? Are they distorted in some way? "Assess whether you are being unnecessarily hard on yourself or other people". (Page 119).

5. Take time out.

6. Control you use of imagination.

7. Learn better ways to communicate.

8. Use logical consequences with others.

9. Learn how to handle criticism and unreasonable demands.

~~~

Part 4: Diet and emotional arousal

Copyright © Jim Byrne 2016

Chapter 14: Dr Jim's Stress and Anxiety Diet

1. Preamble

This information is intended for *educational* purposes only, and does not purport to be medical advice. Bear in mind that each individual body is probably pretty unique, because of its unique nutritional journey through life. So it seems unlikely that we could ever produce a 'universally valid' diet! But it is certainly true that some foods are simply bad for us, causing blood-glucose problems, inflammation problems, and stress-hormone problems, all of which can and will have negative effects upon our mood and emotions: including anger. (But see also Appendix E, section E12, below).

We are changed by the foods we eat, and some experts would say we 'are what we eat'. There are many expert nutritionists available today, at reasonable fees; and you would be well advised to see a nutritionist, or other medical practitioner if you are concerned there might be a link between your current emotional state and your diet.

2. Personal experience of diet and emotional distress

Whereas Renata Taylor-Byrne has formally studied diet and nutrition at diploma level, I (Jim Byrne) got involved in researching my own diet, and its effects upon my body-mind, because of an illness I had developed.

Between 1970 and 1976, I was married to a woman who had studied biochemistry, and also took some training as a cordon beau cook. Therefore, unthinkingly, I was well fed, and kept away from foods that might be bad for my health (by and large!)

In 1976, my first wife and I divorced, and I became a mindless bachelor. I bought only 'convenience foods', and ate out all the time, apart from Sunday lunch, which was a 'family event' with the people with whom I shared a house in Oxford.

Every morning I got up and went to the corner store and bought a pint of milk and a pork pie. (Milk is full of lactic acid, or milk sugar, which selectively feeds our unfriendly gut bacteria, including Candida Albicans. And pork pies are made from pig meat, and pigs are pumped full of antibiotics to prevent diseases in the herd; but those same antibiotics, in my gut, killed off my *friendly* bacteria).

My lunches varied (though I did have a lot of eggs; and non-organic eggs contain a lot of antibiotics, which kill off *friendly* gut bacteria, and allow for Candida overgrowth. They also contain a lot of arachidonic acid (a variety of omega-6 fatty acids, which causes inflammation; while organic eggs are high in omega-3 fatty acids, which quell inflammation. And inflammation is a cause of physical and emotional health problems).

Every evening I had the same thing for my dinner/tea: 'Bhuna Chicken'. (Bhuna chicken was sold in the Bengali restaurant down the road from where I lived. It was made from factory-farmed chicken, which is full of antibiotics, to prevent diseases killing off the flock; but the same antibiotics, in my guts, killed off what was left of my friendly bacteria, and allowed unfriendly bacteria – like Candida Albicans – to flourish. And the most prominent taste of the Bhuna chicken was sweetness: from the handfuls of sugar in which it was cooked. And sugar is a neurotoxin, which suppressed my immune system for hours after eating it).

After one year of living like this, I went to work in Bangladesh. Firstly, I had to submit to a range of vaccinations, each of which probably impaired my immune system (and I have since worked with a homeopath to reverse some of that damage!) Then, upon arriving in Bangladesh, I hired a cook, who fed me rice three times per day. Sweet Bengali Pudding, for breakfast; rice with curried vegetables, and polluted river prawns for lunch; rice with curried vegetables, and polluted river prawns for evening meal; followed by a sweet. Yes: Sweet Bengali Pudding!

After one year in Bangladesh, I had a massive allergic reaction. My body became covered with hot hives. Even my tongue and eyeballs were erupting with urticaria. Some friends and I were on a steam-boat, half way to Khulna, and the boat would not turn back. So we had to travel to Khulna, stay overnight, and then take the first steam-boat back to Dhaka the following day. By the time I arrived in Dhaka, I was delirious. My friends took me to a private doctor (British trained!) I believe the doctor panicked, and instead of placing me under observation for twenty-four hours, and doing some proper diagnostic tests, he simply got a big hypodermic syringe, sucked some antibiotic into it; followed by adrenaline; and then some cortisol. And he pumped this concoction into my right hip.

I was high as a kite for days. I felt like god. But when I came down my energy was half what it had been; and I had permanent dhobi itch; or what the Americans call jock itch; and indeed, on very hot and humid days, I got intense itchiness in all moist parts of my body. My mood was also lower than it had been.

It took three or four years for me to learn that this is a problem called 'systemic Candidiasis', which most western doctors did not understand at that time, and perhaps that has not change much (for all I now know). This condition is perhaps now included under the newer heading of 'dysbiosis', or imbalanced or unbalanced gut flora and fauna.

Fortunately, I got some advice from the late Kevin Benson, a specialist in herbal remedies, at *Food Therapy*, in Halifax, in 1981, or '82. I learned that the Candida spore has a negative effect upon our body and mind, and it's normally held in check by our friendly gut bacteria. We need to reduce sugar and yeast in our diets, and to take an anti-fungal substance (caprylic acid), and also to supplement with friendly bacteria, like Acidophilus Bifidus, and others. I also read a book by Leon Chaitow on the nature of Candida Albicans, and how to control it using dietary restrictions[110]. That was the beginning of my journey into researching the effects of gut bacteria on health, including mood and emotion. (See Jacobs, 1994; and Trowbridge and Walker, 1989)[111].

Because I was sensitized to the gut-brain-mind connection through my personal experience of diet and ill health, I was alert to new research coming out about similar unconventional insights; including the information that trans-fats are linked to problems of lack of control of anger[112]; and research showing that British prisoners who were switched to a diet high in omega-3 fatty acids experienced a reduction in aggressive incidents, fights, etc., with their fellow prisoners.

I then, also found that I occasionally got a depressed or anxious client who had no apparent psychological problem as the cause or stimulus for their condition, but who was on a high sugar and yeast diet, and who was, in fact, suffering the effects of Candida Albicans overgrowth. Once they changed their diets, their depression and anxiety problems cleared up.

So I learned about the gut-brain-mind connection the hard way; the personal way; and I also collected empirical evidence of the truth of those insights from my counselling practice!

3. No universal agreement regarding diet

As far as I can tell, after years of personal research, there is no universal agreement about the precise kind of diet which will promote or reduce stress, although we have some pretty good ideas of some of the major culprits, and some of the main forms of 'best practice'.

As suggested by many other sources of advice, it is advisable to eat lots of fresh fruit and vegetables (if you know you can *tolerate* the fruit!). And, actually, this guideline should be expressed the other way around: Eat *lots of vegetables* and *less* fruit. Fruits contain sugars, and even though they are 'natural sugars', they can still cause problems for our blood-sugar management system. So do not over-consume them. (High GI [glycaemic index] foods push our blood sugar levels too high. See section 4[b] above).

Sugars also occur naturally in vegetables, and some people are so sensitive to sugars that they have to reduce their consumption of those vegetables which are highest in such elements as fructans, oligosaccharides, disaccharides, monosaccharaides, and polyols. These elements are normally referred to by the acronym of FodMaps; and there are some online information sites regarding the nature of FodMaps, and which foods contain them.

4. Schools of thought on diet

There are many schools of thought on diet and health; perhaps several dozen; or even more. There are many different types of diet in circulation today. (See section 3 of Part 1, above, for more detail). Vegetarian diets; the Atkins, Ketogenic and Paleo diets (high in meat and fats, and low in carbs); Semi-vegetarian diets; raw-food diets; wholefood diets; macrobiotic (beans) diet; Weight control diets; Low-calorie diets; high calorie diets; Very low calorie diets; Low-carbohydrate diets; high carb diets; Low-fat diets; high fat diets; crash diets; detox diets. And, of course, the *Metabolic typing diet* ([Atkinson, 2008, pages 50-54]: which I tried but found both unhelpful to me, and difficult to implement).

Dr Atkinson's general (non-metabolic typing) advice is probably sound: He suggests that we:

#Avoid trans-fatty acids (found in junk foods);

minimize (meaning 'eat in moderation') saturated fats (found in meat, dairy, (organic) eggs and seafood products); avoid refined carbohydrates (like white bread, white rice, white pasta, cakes, biscuits, sweets, bottles of juice and pop drinks, and most breakfast cereals);

avoid sugar (including the sugars found in junk and processed foods);

avoid artificial sweeteners;

avoid refined soya products (because refined soya is [no joke!] seen as unfit for feeding to piglets, as it damages their guts!)

restrict salt consumption to six grams (or one-eighth of an ounce) per day;

avoid or limit mercury-laden fish. (The only really safe fish that is left on the planet is Wild Alaskan salmon!) Occasional sardines, or a piece of white fish may be tolerable, but levels of pollution are very high indeed! And some people suffer from adult-onset fish-allergy, which is visible on their skin, but most likely also affects their moods and emotions. So do not overdo the fish consumption. To fish meals per week is probably optimal.

Eat at least five portions of vegetables and fruit per day (seven or eight would be better!) But again, there are no 'totally safe' foods. Some vegetables contain high levels of various *sugars* (fructans, oligosaccharides, disaccharides, monosaccharides and polyols [collectively called FODMAPS]); and others contain excessive amounts of *lectins*; both of which can cause inflammation in the bowel

Drink filtered water – at least six to eight glasses per day, to stay hydrated.

Eat as much of your food from organic sources as possible.

And, take nutritional supplements, including a complete multivitamin complex, B-complex, omega-3 fatty acid supplement (like krill oil or cod liver oil); and friendly gut bacteria (like Acidophilus).

"Your health and mood is intimately linked to the food choices that you make". Dr Mark Atkinson (2008)

~~~

There is *no universal agreement* about what works for anybody, and some researchers now believe that a diet has to be personalized to the individual, because we each have an individual history of environmental effects which impact our genes.

Many experts recommend the ***Mediterranean diet*** - high in vegetables, fish and olive oil, and low in meat consumption[113]. See, for example: www.nhs.uk/Livewell/Goodfood/Pages/what-is-a-Mediterranean-diet.aspx.

Or (occasionally, but *not* long-term) the ***Paleo diet*** - high in meat, fish, vegetables, fruit; and excluding (most) grains and dairy. See: thepaleodiet.com/what-to-eat-on-the-Paleo-diet/)[114]. (But this diet probably involves eating too much meat, according to Dr Michael Greger, 2016). Meat contains the essential fatty acid (omega-6), but it seems from Dr Greger's argument that we should not have too much of this fatty acid – even though it's essential. It seems we need to watch the ratio of omega-3 to omega-6. (See Simopoulos, 2002)[115]. So the emerging Nordic diet may be worth considering; or the Mediterranean diet, because they both favour fish over meat, with the Nordic involving more fish.

Eating organic foods is one way of minimizing the chemical pollutants that get into our bodies and impair our ability to function healthily in the face of the pressures and strains of daily life, according to Bart Cunningham, PhD.[116] There is also recent research which suggests a link between trans-fats (including hydrogenated fats in processed foods) and aggression, irritability and impatience.[117]

5. Stress management advice

The Stress Management Society gives the following advice: "*If you want a strong nervous system, boost your intake of vitamins B, C and E, together with minerals magnesium and zinc. The best source of these nutrients is from food, rather than supplements. So eat a balanced diet of meat, nuts, seeds, fresh fruit and vegetables and oily fish. If you need to snack during the day, try pumpkin or sunflower seeds and fruit, particularly (greenish) bananas. Fresh organic food is the best source. If you can't get fresh, frozen vegetables are a reasonable alternative as much of their nutritional content is retained.*" [118]

We suggest you follow most of this advice, except for the supplementation of vitamins and minerals. Unless you are on a wholly organic diet, your food will be largely denatured and devoid of much nutritional value; you may not know what to eat in order to have 'a balanced diet'; and it you cook your food, you will lose some of the nutrients that are in it; therefore you need to use vitamin and mineral supplements of a good, natural-source quality.

The Stress Management Society also rightly emphasizes the importance of drinking lots of water over the course of the day: "*If you want to deal with stress, drink water. It hydrates every part of the body and brain and helps you to better cope with stressful situations. A good rule is to take a few sips every 15 minutes. The best source is room-temperature still water bought in glass bottles (some plastic bottles can leach chemicals into the water inside) or use a jug filter system that you fill from the tap.*" (Stress Management Society, 2012/2016).

6. Proportions of food groups

How much protein, carbohydrate and other foods should we eat? There is a lot of emphasis today on having five (six, or seven) portions per day of fruit and vegetables. Before that particular campaign began, the Department of Health (in Britain) and many nutritionists were recommending that about fifty to seventy percent of our daily intake of food should come from complex carbohydrate, such as brown rice, pasta, wholemeal bread, millet, potatoes, and so on. (And this kind of ratio is maintained in the US to this day). About twenty-five percent (they said) should be unsaturated fats, from sources like oily fish, nuts, seeds, cold-pressed oils, like olive oil, flaxseed oil, and so on.

And ideally you need about fifteen percent of your food intake to be in the form of protein sources such as grass fed meat, (especially liver); fish (especially oily varieties [which contain more omega-3 fatty acid], though some white fish is very good for the brain); and eggs (preferably organic free range). Keep the meat proportion low and the fish proportion high, to reduce the omega-6/omega-3 ratio (Simopoulos, 2002).

Increasingly, we see recommendations that about 80% of your dinner plate should be vegetables, with a small amount of protein. Or, in the case of current UK guidelines: 35% grains and legumes; 35% vegetables and fruit; and the remaining 30% split into three groups: milk and dairy foods (10%); meat, fish and alternatives (10%); and foods containing fat, and foods containing sugar (10%).

The best and safest sources of protein are probably wild Pacific salmon, or wild Alaskan salmon; grass fed lamb; organic, free range chicken; and organic eggs.

7. Food combining, or not

Some theorists believe that combining complex carbohydrates with a protein can reduce stress and provide a solid fuel for daily energy requirements: (Atkinson, 2008: page 57). This, however, contradicts the *Hay Diet*, which recommends keeping carbohydrates and proteins separate, in meals separated by at least four hours! (However, there does not seem to be any scientific studies supporting the Hay approach to food combining – although Renata and I have found it very helpful in reducing indigestion, and promoting efficient elimination).

Others argue that too much carbohydrate, especially refined forms, could cause stress (e.g. Gangwisch, J. et al. (2015) in *ScienceDaily*, 2015)[119]. On the other hand, oily fish, like salmon, mackerel and sardines, with green vegetables and complex carbohydrate are believed to be particularly beneficial. There *are* scientific studies to support the claims about the impact of oily fish on the reduction of panic attacks. For example, Perretta, 2001, page 90).[120]

Cunningham (2001) maintains that fast foods, which are normally high in fats and sugars "...*are stressful to our systems*". (Page 201)[121]. So eliminating fast foods would seem like a sensible precaution as part of a stress management programme. And getting rid of sugar and salt in general from our diets is sometimes said to be a good idea, though some theorists think *a small amount of salt* is needed by the body to function normally. In general, however, western diets are overloaded with salt and sugar, and a vast reduction seems to be called for, as high blood sugar levels are bad for stress levels, and high salt levels are implicated in heart attacks and strokes (according to some experts, and some studies). And caffeine, sugar and alcohol are stressful to the body-brain-mind.

The **Ph Diet** is an interesting one, which emphasizes the general guideline that about 75% of the content of each main meal should comprise vegetables. Pasta, rice and potatoes should never be taken as more than a *small* side dish! Avoid pizzas, burgers and other processed foods. Additionally, as Nicki Woodward writes: "*Acidifying foods should be reduced in the diet as much as possible*". According to C Vasey, author of The

Acid-Alkaline Diet... *"These foods are primarily rich in proteins, carbohydrates and/or fats. Cheese, vegetable oils, hard animal fats, bread, pasta, white sugar all fall into this category"*.[122] Sugar and sugary foods are bad; avoid processed foods (especially pastries, pastas and white bread); salt; and minimize saturated dietary fat (as in meat, cheese and eggs).

~~~

8. Drinks and drinking

As a general rule, we can definitely say that you could benefit from minimizing your consumption of caffeine (coffee, tea, cocoa, and cola drinks). Also, avoid sugary drinks (like colas, sodas, pops and power drinks/energy drinks). All of these drinks tend to stoke the build-up of anxiety. And avoid alcohol, if you have Candida overgrowth problems. And minimize it otherwise, which means about one unit of alcohol three times per week. Preferably red wine with a meal.

Green tea is good for you. Camomile tea is very calming of the central nervous system.

Minimize milk, as it contains high levels of lactic acid, which is a sugar that feeds candida, and thus triggers depressed feelings. (Very little research has been done, apparently, on the effect of milk upon the emotional states of *adult* humans. However, a significant degree of research has been done on the effect of milk, via migraine reactions, on *children's moods and behaviours*, and the effects can be quite negative and disruptive of brain-mind functioning)[123].

It is important to drink at least six or eight glasses of water per day, preferably mineral water, or a combination of mineral water and filtered water. (Tap water is bad for your health, because of various forms of pollution, like heavy metals and agricultural chemical run-off).

Avoid sugary cola and pop drinks. And minimize alcohol consumption, as suggested above. (Alcohol can trigger anger, aggression, and suicidal ideation and self-harm acts; and it feeds the unfriendly bacterium, Candida Albicans). Perhaps one unit of alcohol three times per week might be tolerable (especially a red wine). More than that and you will damage your health. Alcohol is a depressant which also disturbs your sleep, which has a negative effect upon your mood the following day. Some nutritionists are concerned that 'green smoothies', or regular 'fruit smoothies' may be bad for us, because they give us a quick spike of sugar (fructose and other forms) which raises our stress level. (For example: Dr Thomas Campbell recommends that you, *"Use your mouth and your teeth the way nature intended and put the smoothies aside or have them just as treats."* [124]

9. Fats and oils

Fats are one of the three macronutrients, which are essential for physical and mental health. The other two are protein and carbohydrates. We also need two micronutrients: vitamins and minerals. And we need water.

We need fat for current energy needs; plus energy storage (for later use); and for the building and rebuilding of our cells, including our brain cells; and to produce myelin, which is essential for transmitting signals from brain cell to brain cell. And certain essential fatty acids (EFA's) are important for brain and emotional health.

But even though we need fat, we can also have *too much*.

Most of the important questions about fat remain unanswered (according to Campbell and Campbell, 2006). The 'diet wars' are as much about fat as any other macronutrient or food group.

Butter is probably quite bad for you (because it is 100% animal fat, and animal fat (and animal-based foods in general) are bad for our general health [according to the China Study, by Campbell and Campbell, 2006]). And margarine is even worse (even though it is vegetable fat – and even though vegetable fat tends to promote health while animal fat reduces it [Campbell and Campbell, 2006: pages 66, and 129-130]). And the reason for the problem with margarine is the chemicals that are used to harden it and colour and flavour it. Most margarines are made from, or contain, trans-fatty acids, which are bad for your body and brain. Some of the chemical processes used in the manufacture of margarine (like bleaching!) are clearly not good for human health! (Source: The Real Food Guide (2017)) [125].

A McDonald's Double Cheeseburger is 67% animal fat, and whole cow's milk is 64% animal fat. Very small amounts of animal fat are probably going to be okay, but we have to keep it low. (Campbell and Campbell, 2006).

So small amounts of extra virgin olive oil dribbled on your (gluten free) bread might be better (as demonstrated by the Mediterranean diet), but keep the quantity to about one teaspoon per day, as processing fats uses up your body's water content, which results in dehydration. (You could also try Extra Virgin Coconut Oil, which is solid at room temperature, and can be spread like butter. [However, Patrick Holford recommends cold-pressed seed oils, like flaxseed oil or hemp oil]. But, again, watch out for dehydration by keeping oil consumption low [or you could significantly increase your water consumption?!]).

Avoid all trans-fats, which are found in junk foods, processed food, and most take-way foods. (See Part 1 of this book, section 4(a), above).

According to Campbell and Campbell (2006), we should probably keep our total fat consumption below 30% (although this has not been established as a 'vital threshold'). It is also difficult for us to figure out how much fat we are eating in any case! It's not easy, since all of the main food groups, in the UK National Food Guide, and the US Food Guide Pyramid (renamed My-Pyramid), contain some fat. So, as a general guideline, it is probably best to keep your animal product consumption low, since there is *a strong parallel between increasing animal products and increasing total fat consumption*. And there is also a strong link between increasing the consumption of animal products and increasing disease! (Campbell and Campbell, 2006: page 83, and page 129-130).

We recommend that you keep your dairy products and meat consumption low or very low. You should probably aim for less than 10% of your total calorie consumption from this food group. (You will still be getting plant based fats from the other food groups, and plant based fats are probably better [based on the results of the China Study]).

Make sure you get at least as much omega-3 fatty acid as omega-6. Again this is difficult to calculate and maintain, because most of our foods contain lots of omega-6 fatty acids, and very few contain much omega-3. The best way to do this is to eat oily fish (like salmon, mackerel, tuna and sardines) at least twice each week. And eat lots of nuts and seeds on a regular basis. Since it is very difficult to measure the fats we are eating, it is probably best to choose a good, healthy, balanced diet, like the Mediterranean or the Nordic diets, and stick to those general guidelines. Perhaps also get cookbooks for those diets, and try to be guided by the types of food recommend therein. (But mainly go for plant based foods, and keep meat and dairy products very low).

What about other uses of oils in the kitchen?

For salad dressings, it is probably best to use olive oil.

And what about frying? We tend not to fry anything. I (Jim) usually poach our salmon fillets, in herb-flavoured water, instead of frying them.

But what do the experts say? One BBC blog reported on some recent frying experiments (by Professor Martin Grootveld, at De Montford University) like this: *'Firstly, try to do less frying, particularly at high temperature. If you are frying, minimise the amount of oil you use, and also take steps to remove the oil from the outside of the fried food, perhaps with a paper towel.*

'To reduce aldehyde (which are noxious chemical products of the frying process) go for an oil or fat high in monounsaturated or saturated lipids (preferably greater than 60% for one or the other, and more than 80% for the two combined), and low in polyunsaturates (less than 20%).

'He thinks the ideal "compromise" oil for cooking purposes is olive oil,

> *"because it is about 76% monounsaturates, 14% saturates and only 10% polyunsaturates - monounsaturates and saturates are much more resistant to oxidation (which produces trans-fats) than are polyunsaturates".'*
> (Source: Mosley, M., 2015)[126].

If we (Renata and Jim) - very occasionally - fry anything, then we add some butter to the olive oil, which is even better at resisting the oxidation process (which is what produces the aldehydes). And rapeseed oil and goose fat were also found by Prof Grootveld's study to resist the oxidation process (and thus produced a healthier friend food result).

10. Never skip breakfast

Don't skip your breakfast, no matter how late or busy you might be, as you need a solid supply of *food-derived-glucose*, **burning slowly** throughout the morning, to keep your blood sugar level at a suitable and fairly constant level. Porridge or cooked fish make a good, slow-burning breakfast; or wholemeal brown toast and organic eggs. Make sure you eat at least three nutritious meals every day; and have a light snack mid-morning and mid-afternoon, to keep your blood sugar level up. Always eat in a relaxing environment. And avoid simple sugars, as they are seen to over-boost blood sugar levels, precipitating insulin release, and a quick fall back in blood sugar levels, thus reducing energy, concentration, and potentially boosting stress levels via the release of adrenaline.

Some people are so sensitive to sugar that they cannot even cope well with fruit sugar, and those individuals fare better on a diet of seven portions of vegetables per day, and no fruit at all.

The worst kind of breakfast is no breakfast at all!

The next worse kind of breakfasts is one of refined carbohydrate and simple sugars, such as white toast, or any kind of bread made from refined flour; sugary cereals; jams and marmalades; and so on.

The best kind of breakfast (according to some theorists) consists of complex carbohydrate, such as porridge or muesli, combined with a couple of pieces of fresh fruit (if you can tolerate the fructose), such as apples or bananas. (However, in relation to carbohydrate consumption, watch out for *gluten intolerance* in yourself - and it is advisable to only eat gluten-free breakfast cereals (complex, not refined or processed). Also watch out for food intolerances - allergic reactions - and eliminate those foods to which you are currently allergic). You can always consult a nutritional therapist regarding what to eat for your particular needs and problems.

A couple of times per week, a protein breakfast would be good, such as grilled mackerel, kippers, or traditional (organic) bacon and egg, etc. It is best to eat like a "king/queen" at breakfast, to fuel your morning's work. Then have a reasonable lunch, to carry you through the afternoon. And finally, have a light meal in the evening.

PS: Actually, for several months now, I have been having salad for breakfast, with nuts and seeds and some low-sugar berries. And I seem to be thriving on that!

11. Snacks, supplements and raw food

Mid-morning and mid-afternoon, it is important to have both (small) snacks and (10 minute) naps. The best forms of snacks are probably a handful of nuts or seeds, and a piece of fruit, with a bottle of mineral water or a herbal tea. Brazil nuts are particularly high in selenium and magnesium, which are both calming. Dr John Briffa believes that just three or four Brazil nuts per day can stabilize the moods of anxious individuals.[127]

If you prefer to take a magnesium supplement, then 400 milligrams per day is probably a good level to take. Some theorists believe milk is particularly helpful, because its calcium content is calming. However, it also contains lactose, which is a form of sugar, and it has been shown to cause emotional problems (Brown, 2017); so watch the consumption level. And the Paleo theorists think dairy products cause inflammation in the guts, which can then cause mood swings. (80 or 90% of the serotonin in our bodies is, apparently, produced in our guts!) There is no doubt that many people are lactose intolerant, and we have included a reference to research that shows milk can have a negative impact on mood, emotions and behaviours in children, and, by implication, in adults also.

Raw food is very important, as much cooked food is very low in nutritional content, and especially enzymes, which are essential for digestion: so at least one salad meal per day would seem to be sensible. Furthermore, eating lots of salad vegetables seems like a good idea. The Chinese would not agree with that, as they think the digestion process is aided by lightly stir-frying vegetables.

~~~

12. Find out for yourself

However there really is no alternative to experimenting with these ideas, and trying to map the effects of particular kinds of food on your energy level and your mood. We do know from scientific studies that caffeine and alcohol are particular causes of concern, in that they stimulate the sympathetic nervous system, pushing your stress level up, causing irritability and anger, anxiety, panic attacks, depression and insomnia. (Perretta, 2001, page 88)[128].

Smoking also tends to increase stress levels, and some recreational drugs are also stressors.   Therefore, many alternative health practitioners and nutritionists advocate giving up smoking; reducing alcohol consumption; avoiding stimulants; and restricting your intake of caffeine to two cups of fresh ground coffee per day, or four cups of tea. (Cunningham, 2001). Dr John Briffa recommends *complete elimination* of caffeine for individuals who are *"on the anxious side"*. We recommend that you reduce or eliminate smoking; alcohol consumption; and breathing polluted air.

Most practitioners recommend consuming less than two units of alcohol every other day, as a maximum, for men, and half of that for women; and also slowly getting off tobacco completely.   Marijuana has also been implicated in the causation of panic attacks and paranoia.

13. Supplements and healthy foods

Because modern methods of agriculture have resulted in reduced levels of nutrition in our foods, and many of these foods are further denatured by the food-processing industry, you are strongly advised to take a good quality multivitamin and mineral supplement, plus a full spectrum B-complex, including B5 and B2; iron, magnesium and calcium.

You will also benefit from extra vitamin C (at least one gram per day). Perretta (2001) recommends the following foods in particular: avocado; mushrooms; spring greens and spinach; liver; millet; guava and papaya. And a friendly bacteria supplement will support your gut health.

14. Finale

Green vegetables are recommended by many nutritionists, and the British Department of Health. And don't forget the oily fish! It aids all brain functions, including managing stress. Best oily fish: Wild Alaskan salmon, (or Wild Pacific salmon) which is available fresh (chilled) or in tins at Marks and Spencer, UK; tinned sardines, which can be with tomato sauce for taste purposes; grilled fresh mackerel; or trout.

And finally, lettuce is a natural tranquillizer[129], so it seems sensible to eat lots of it; and drinking Chamomile tea may also calm the nervous system, and reduce insomnia[130]. But be careful. Everything we put in our digestive system has the potential to produce side-effects; and some investigators have reported anecdotal evidence that Chamomile tea can interfere with antidepressant medication! (See 'Health Unblocked' blog[131]). (Not that we can recommend antidepressant medication, which seems to be no better than a placebo, and has some very nasty side effects which will, predictably, affect a high proportion of the users of these drugs. 'Food is the best medicine'!)

~~~

If you want to check out the areas of agreement and disagreement among medical practitioners on the subject of diet and emotional wellbeing, then take a look at this debate: 'Sugar, Gluten, Paleo, Vegan: 3 Doctors Debate The Best Way To Eat', here: http://www.mindbodygreen.com/ revitalize/ video/sugar-gluten-paleo-vegan-3-doctors- debate-the-best-way-to-eat

And remember: This is not *medical* advice. It is *educational* information. For medical advice, please see your medical practitioner, GP, DO, or holistic, complementary or alternative health physician; or your health coach. For professional advice and help with your diet, please see a registered nutritional therapist or nutritionist.

~~~

Appendix A: The importance of diet, exercise and sleep in managing your anger problems

By Renata Taylor-Byrne and Jim Byrne, 2019

~~~

This appendix presents some extracts from two of our earlier books - Byrne (2018)[132] and Taylor-Byrne (2017)[133] - on the links between diet, exercise and sleep, on the one hand, and anger, on the other.

A1: Managing anger with diet and nutrition

In Taylor-Byrne and Byrne (2017), we explored - among other things - the key ways in which *diet can influence anger.* Some of the key findings were as follows:

Firstly, (unlike in the case of depression) there is at least one study which supports the idea that there is a link between low serotonin levels and the expression of anger, annoyance and irritation (specifically, low serotonin was linked to a reduced ability to self-manage rising levels of anger). We also presented evidence which showed that 5HTP, a natural nutritional supplement (from a West African medicinal plant called *Griffonia simpicifolia*), can be effective in restoring serotonin, an important neurotransmitter within the brain, thus reducing the expression of angry and hostile behaviour, as evidenced by Julie Ross's (2002) case study example[134].

The levels of copper and manganese in the client's body can have an effect on levels of anger; so vitamin and mineral supplementation seems to be important to address.

The link between violent behaviour - by young offenders (in prison) - and the condition known as 'reactive hypoglycaemia' (where blood sugar levels fall too low after eating high carbohydrate meals [because the body overacts and – in sugar-induced crisis - mops up too much of the sugar]) - has been established by scientific research. There is thus an obvious connection between fluctuating blood sugar levels and anger management problems, and this can guide us in recommending particular (low sugar, slow-burning) foods to our angry clients.

A number of studies have established a definite link between a reduction in the consumption of sugar and refined foods, (on the one hand), and anger and anti-social behaviour, (on the other). In a similar vein, reductions in diets containing trans-fats, mainly involving hydrogenated fats in processed foods, led to a reduction in impatience, irritability and aggression in research participants.

Conversely, the link between pro-social behaviour and a healthy diet has also been evidenced by research. Dietary changes which increase the nutritional content of people's diets (especially introducing omega-3 fatty acids, as found for example in oily fish; plus vitamin and mineral supplements) result in improvements in pro-social behaviour, and better emotion and mood control. Anger levels declined in prisoners whose diet had been supplemented with fish oils, vitamins and minerals: and it has been shown that omega-3 fats have a rapid and significant impact on aggression in children and adults.

~~~

Let us expand somewhat our consideration of the connection between _anger_ and diet: Anger is affected by nutrition to a surprising extent, which is confirmed by the research findings of Dr Julia Ross (2002).

Ross is a psychotherapist and director of Recovery Systems, a clinic in California that treats mood, eating and addiction problems with nutritional therapy and biochemical rebalancing. And her findings are mirrored by the research findings of Patrick Holford (Chief Executive of the Food for the Brain Foundation, in the UK, and a leading nutrition expert)[135].

Both of these experts quote research results which show that angry, aggressive behaviour can originate from chemical imbalances in the body, and they give examples of aggressive behaviour being transformed when nutrients were given to people suffering from low levels of serotonin or who were suffering from hypoglycaemia. For example, there were some astonishing results from the work done by Professor Stephen Schoenthaler, with 3,000 prison inmates in California in 1983[136]. There was a massive reduction in aggressive behaviour when the research study participants, the inmates, were given a diet which was stripped of refined food and sugar.

Schoenthaler's research findings were later replicated in a double-blind study of 1,482 juveniles and several follow-up studies confirmed his findings, which revealed strong, unequivocal evidence of the link between anger and aggression, on the one hand, and the consumption of sugar, processed food and transfats, on the other.

And in the UK, between 1995 and 1997, at Aylesbury Young Offenders Institution, a placebo-controlled, randomised trial, was conducted by Dr Bernard Gesch (2002), in which young offenders were given food supplements (including vitamins, minerals and essential fatty acids), and it was found that they committed 37% fewer violent offences, while the inmates who received the placebo showed no such reduction; thus demonstrating that improved nutrition reduces angry outbursts (which were being fuelled by vitamin and mineral and fatty acid deficiencies)[137].

The whole range of research studies, described in Taylor-Byrne and Byrne (2017), point out the relationship between the body and its reaction to:

(1) Toxins in the diet - like alcohol, caffeine and trans-fats – and also:

(2) The negative effects of nutritional deficiencies (such as lack of omega-3 fatty acids, vitamins and minerals), and/or:

(3) Blood-sugar dysregulation...

...in these cases resulting in anger and anti-social behaviour; but also potentially playing a role in anxiety and depression.

~~~

For further information, please see Appendix E, Section E12.

~~~

A2: How anger can be reduced by exercise:

According to the British National Health Service website, anger is effectively reduced in intensity by exercising, including walking, swimming and yoga. Research studies have supported this view, and here are some examples which have provided valuable evidence on the role of exercise in anger reduction:

Research conducted by Joseph Tkacz, *et al.*, (2008), found that aerobic exercise regimes reduced anger expression among obese children[138]. It was the first study which had been conducted to assess the value of having structured aerobic exercise sessions for overweight children, and the findings pointed to the value of exercise sessions after school.

Also, there was a study which investigated levels of anger amongst undergraduates at the University of Georgia. It looked at whether physical education (exercise) could moderate anger: (Reynolds, 2010); and it was reported in the *New York Times* magazine[139].

The 16 students selected were regularly oversensitive to provocations, and their anger was easily triggered. They were subjected to different research conditions (*provocations*), designed to arouse their anger.

Firstly, those provocations were experienced without the benefits of exercise; Secondly, they were experienced after the benefits of exercise.

The research results revealed that, the provocations had a stronger angering effect – producing a higher level of anger - *before* the exercise than they did after the participants had engaged in physical exercise.

After they had exercised, they were able to show composure and self-assurance in the face of emotional provocation. The physical exercise program did reduce their levels of anger, prompting the lead researcher, Nathaniel Thoms, a stress physiologist, to say:

"Exercise, even a single bout of it, can have a robust prophylactic (therapeutic) effect against the build-up of anger…it's like taking an aspirin to combat heart disease. You reduce your risk".

This result is echoed by the advice of the Mayo Clinic Staff, who have written that the higher the levels of stress a person is experiencing, the more likely they are to have high levels of anger, and that these effects can be diminished by vigorous and pleasurable exercise.

For further information, please see Taylor-Byrne and Byrne (2017), for more specific information on research into different forms of exercise.

~~~

A3. Sleep

Sleep is hugely important for our physical and mental health.

You need to aim to get 7.5 to 9 hours of sleep every single night, without exception; and preferably normally more than eight hours.

If you have sleep problems, do not take sleeping pills, as that will prevent you having proper, restful sleep, and the kind of sleep during which you not only process the stresses and strains of the day, but physically clean out the debris from your brain.

If you suffer from insufficient sleep, you will not be able to maintain the level of physical and mental health needed to sustain happy and successful relationships at home and in work and in the wider world. (See Chapter 5 of Byrne, 2018)[140]. In particular, your emotional intelligence will decline, and you will be more prone to angry outbursts, which are the kiss of death to all relationships.

According to Gordon (2013)[141]:

"Both correlational and experimental ... evidence suggest that when people are sleep deprived, they feel more *irritable, angry* and *hostile*".

Like other emotional problems, the causation of anger tends to be multi-factorial; it comes from many supplementary sources; like diet, exercise, sleep deprivation; and poor stress management in general. A blog post by 'My-Sahana' cites nine sources of anger-inducing problems, of which lack of sleep is one:

"Not sleeping enough can result in feeling edgy and easily irritable. Chronic insomnia, sleep apnoea or other sleep disorders can be linked to recurrent bouts of anger". My-Sahana (2012)[142].

~~~

In Chapter 14 of her latest book, due for publication soon, Renata Taylor-Byrne presents some additional information about the link between insufficient sleep, on the one hand, and anger problems, on the other[143].

This is what she writes there:

The connection between lack of sleep and a high level of anger is so apparent that it has led to the nickname "Slanger," which is described as the seething anger that consumes a sleep-deprived person. This is described in an article in the *Daily Mail* newspaper, on the 14th January 2016, by Helen Carroll, entitled: *"How losing sleep can turn women into MONSTERS:* Subtitle: *It's known as sleep anger - or 'slanger'. And as these mothers confess, its toll on your family can be devastating."*[144]

The article describes the experiences of three women, from different professional backgrounds, whose problems with anger could be traced back to lack of sleep the night before an anger-inducing incident. One of the three women stated that she needed ten hours of sleep each night to avoid using angry and aggressive behaviour with her family members. In one incident, where she was suffering the effects of a lack of sleep after a Halloween party, she smashed her husband's iPad during an argument.

She could identify the start of her angry behaviour during the early months of her baby's night feeding, when her sleep would be regularly broken.

The same experience led another mother to resolve to not have any more children. The third mother described being sent on a negotiations skills course after she had only six hours sleep and she exploded at her colleagues during a business meeting. She had a similar experience after her mother's death, when she was suffering from lack of sleep. She threw cutlery at family members during a discussion. They were aware that lack of sleep affected her in this way and accepted her heartfelt apology after she had experienced a good night's sleep.

There are different explanations for *why* people become angry through lack of sleep, and Dr Irshaad Ebrahim, based at the London Sleep Centre, considers that if we have insufficient sleep, then our bodies are unable to process certain chemicals which the body needs, in order to function properly. One chemical that needs to be processed, serotonin, (which manages our energy levels and moods), is affected by lack of sleep; and for some people they become very annoyed and angry, whilst others retreat into themselves and revert to silence.

An experiment that was conducted by Matthew Walker (2017) and his colleagues gave a clear picture of what happens to people when they are deprived of sleep. The researchers took two groups of people – both groups were composed of young people who did not have any health problems. One group had a good night's sleep, and the other group were instructed to stay awake all night and were monitored throughout the night to make sure they did not sleep.

The following day each of the participants in the two groups had their brains scanned. They were also shown one hundred pictures, with varied content. For example they were shown negative images, such as a snake ready to bite someone, and a house on fire; and pictures with less emotive images such as a piece of driftwood, and a basket. The variety of emotion–evoking pictures gave the experimenters an opportunity to observe the responses of the participants to the increasingly negative images as they occurred.

What the findings showed was that there was a lot of activity in the amygdalas of those participants who were lacking in sleep; (and the amygdala is the brain's panic-button, and it is involved in the management of emotions, especially fear and anger, and it's connected to the autonomic system's 'fight or flight' response). The results of the brain scans showed that there was an increase of *over 60%* in the sleep-deprived participants' emotional reactions to the pictures they were shown (as compared to the reactions of those participants who had not been sleep-deprived). This was the largest reaction that Matthew Walker had seen in all the sleep research he had been conducting.

In complete contrast, the brain scans of the group of participants who had a full night's sleep had a much reduced level of reaction in the amygdala, even though they had seen the same pictures as the sleep deprived group.

Walker (2017) speculated that if we don't have sufficient sleep our brain regresses to a level of primitive functioning, and we can't order information into its proper setting (for example reacting to pictures as if they are the real objects rather than paper representations of them).

He describes witnessing 'pendulum-like' alterations in the emotional states and moods of the sleep deprived participants. The variation in their moods was huge, from over-excitement to destructive anger, in very quick fluctuations of their mood state. He therefore considered that if people are sleep deprived, then they don't *just* suffer from depression and negativity, and stabilise in that state, but that they experience the full range of emotions from extreme happiness to deep, self-destructive feelings of negativity and despair.

Walker wanted to know the reason why, as human beings, we were so vulnerable to over-emotionality when we were short of sleep. So he conducted more studies using the MRI scanner (magnetic-resonance-imager).

He examined the difference in the composition of the pre-frontal cortex[145] of human beings when compared to those of other primates, and found that there is a greater amount of development in that part of the human brain. It is also closely connected to the amygdala (our danger-spotting mechanism), and when human beings are fully rested, he considers that there is a balance between these two parts of our brain. Our pre-frontal cortex moderates inappropriate behaviour by damping down the immediate fear and emotionality of the amygdala.

Without sleep, this balance between these two parts of the brain goes haywire, and this he considered to be an explanation of the over-emotionality and irrationality of the participants' behaviour which he observed in his experiments.

In a blog on the 'Psychology Today' website, there is a post by Romeo Vitelli, entitled, 'Does Lack of Sleep Make People More Violent?' The subtitle is this: 'The link between sleep problems and aggression, and the cost, is becoming clear.[146] (Posted Oct 26, 2016). In his blog, Vitelli summarises the findings of Anne Herlache and Zlatan Krizan of Iowa State University. One of the most significant was that there was a reduction in the violent behaviour of prison inmates when their problems with sleep had been dealt with. Their research also established a connection between an *inability* to curb uninhibited behaviour, and a *lack* of good quality sleep. And they also examined the research into violent behaviour between couples and intimidation between teenagers and children, and found evidence of a definite connection between these behaviours and disturbed, impaired sleep.

~~~

Appendix B: Conflict Styles and Anger Management

By Renata Taylor-Byrne, Copyright (c) November 2018

B1 Introduction

> *"Communication is to relationship what breathing is to living..."*
>
> Virginia Satir (1972/1983)[147]

In this appendix, I want to present a simple quiz that helps us to understand how we handle conflict in our current relationships. This quiz will give you a clear picture of how you deal with pressure in situations of interpersonal conflict.

The related descriptions and explanations will also clarify what is wrong with particular ways of communicating, and which approach to communication is best for the health and happiness of your couple relationship (and indeed of all of your relationships); including the avoidance of inappropriate anger outbursts.

The quiz, created by Virginia Satir (1972/1983), outlines the five main ways of handling conflict with others. Four of these are unhealthy, or unhelpful, and one is healthy, effective and helpful.

Satir created a system of *conjoint-family-therapy*, and was a pioneering therapist who showed that families play a significant part in the development of the problems of individuals, and that blaming individual family members for their problems was unfair, because the problems that counselling and therapy clients showed up with were learned and created in their family of origin.

The helpful thing about this quiz is that it shows you a range of patterns that people play out when they are dealing with interpersonal conflict.

The strategies used vary from constructive to really unhelpful and ineffective.

If you complete the quiz below, and you look at your results, you'll be able to see your current favourite approach, and how to change your behaviour if you are not happy with the result.

B2 Five ways of handling conflict

Here are the five ways of handling conflict which Satir identified:

(1) PLACATING – This involves: Pacifying, calming or appeasing behaviour. (Appeasing means to make someone calm and less hostile by giving in to their demands). The aim here is most obviously to stop the other person becoming, or remaining, angry and aggressive. The placator tends to feel relatively worthless, or weak, and to go along with the idea that their adversary – or the person challenging them - is superior, or significantly stronger, in some way.

Your *'placating'* score shows how much you tend to *placate* or *appease* others to calm them down, instead of dealing with what they are saying, doing or presenting to you. And of course, after placating them for a long time, you may have collected enough 'brown stamps' to cash them in for a really big, loud, angry outburst.

~~~

(2) BLAMING – This approach is about: Holding someone to account, in a *condemning* or *accusatory* way – which is, of course, angry and aggressive behaviour by definition. The aim here is most often to get the other person to regard you as strong; or to deny your own responsibility. The blamer finds fault with others; dictates to them; and is relatively bossy.

Your *'blaming'* score shows how far you are liable to *blame* other people when under stress; and how angry and aggressive you tend to be.

~~~

(3) DISTRACTING – This style of conflict management involves: Diverting, changing the subject, cracking a joke for entertainment, etc. The aim of the distractor is most often to deny the threat by ignoring it; pretending it does not exist.

Your *'distracting'* score shows how much you tend to *distract* yourself and other people from the problems being presented. This is a form of manipulation, which is also part of indirect aggression; and it can also precipitate aggression in those people you try to manipulate or distract.

~~~

(4) COMPUTING – This approach is about: Assessing, analysing, and theorising about what you are experiencing.

The aim here is most often to *deny a felt sense of threat,* and to relate to the problem *as if it was totally harmless.*

It can also be an attempt to restore you sense of self-esteem by using big words and fancy ideas.

Your *'computing'* score shows how far you tend to *cut off from* your feelings.

This is also sometimes called intellectualizing (with the implication that you use intellectualizing when you should be dealing with your feelings!)

In this modality it is difficult to be appropriately assertive with others.

~~~

(5) LEVELLING – Being frank, open, honest, and above board. Telling the truth as you see it. The aim here is most often to be fair, equal and/or *human-growth promoting.*

Your *'levelling'* score shows how far you tend to react *creatively* and *flexibly* and *humanely.*

It is about being reality-oriented, appropriate, and constructive. This is the core of assertive behaviour.

~~~

This quiz tests how you react when life gets difficult: particularly during interpersonal conflict.

B3 The Personal Styles Quiz:

Here is the quiz:

Read through the following list of 20 statements.

Place a tick (☑) against the statement number of any statement with which you *strongly* agree.

(You will need these numbers to mark your resulting score).

Choose *as many statements as you like from the list* if you think they reflect you or your views.

You should choose *at least* seven statements, but more if you like.

❐ 1. Conflict is something I try to reduce as soon as possible.

❐ 2. If someone's going to tell me something I don't want to hear, I'll quickly and smoothly try to change the subject.

❐ 3. Conflict is healthy if it means the people involved solve a problem.

❐ 4. It's important that people know who's responsible for a mistake.

❐ 5. Catching people off-guard with a compliment is a good way to ease tension.

❐ 6. I've been told I can be unemotional.

❐ 7. I've been told that sometimes I let people take me for granted.

❐ 8. I can get stressed but I try not to let it affect my life too much.

❐ 9. Avoiding taking responsibility for my actions is a good way to shift blame.

❐ 10. In the past, I have taken the blame for something when it wasn't my fault.

❒ 11. I can keep my head clear by distancing myself when those around me are getting edgy.

❒ 12. Hopefully, people know that once a conflict with me is finished, we can then move on.

❒ 13. I'll fight my corner at all costs to make sure I can hold my head up high.

❒ 14. I dislike being shouted at, so I'll usually try to soothe the situation.

❒ 15. If I'm clever and funny enough I can keep conflict at bay.

❒ 16. If something bad happens, I cut off from my emotions; it feels safer to not let my guard down.

❒ 17. I'm not scared to confront someone – but I try to do so without making the other person feel bad.

❒ 18. Becoming overly-emotional during conflict is no way to solve problems.

❒ 19. I have a long memory when it comes to remembering others who've crossed me in some way.

❒ 20. If I've forgotten to do something I said I would, some 'social flirting' keeps people off my back.

B4 The quiz mark sheet

Now that you've chosen at least seven statements as being ones that you agree with, take a look at the grid below. Then tick those numbers in that grid that correspond to the statement numbers that you've ticked in the list above:

Tick the option numbers below that you chose above					
	1	4	2	6	3
	7	9	5	11	8
	10	13	15	16	12
	14	19	20	18	17
TOTAL >					
Inter-personal style →	PLACATING	BLAMING	DISTRACTING	COMPUTING	LEVELLING

Next, add up the number of ticks in each column, and place the total in the **TOTAL** row.

~~~

The next table shows a worked example:

Tick the option numbers below that you chose above					
	1	4☑	2☑	6☑	3
	7	9	5☑	11	8
	10☑	13☑	15☑	16	12☑
	14☑	19	20☑	18	17
TOTAL >	2	2	4	1	1
Interpersonal style →	PLACATING	BLAMING	DISTRACTING	COMPUTING	LEVELLING

B5 Scoring

Which column has the highest score? Count the number of ticks (☑) in each column. The one with the *highest score* is your favourite strategy. In the example above, it's the 'Distracting' column.

Which one is highest for your score-grid? Whichever one it is, than that one is your *dominant* conflict management style.

You could also have a 'close second' style, if two scores are close to each other.

In the example in the grid above, we can see that 'distracting' is the style most often chosen by the person who completed that grid, followed by 'placating' and 'blaming'. So this person would be called 'a distractor', as a shorthand description.

B6 Exploring the conflict styles

When things get tough in our lives we choose one or more of these personality patterns. Here is more of an explanation of these styles of behaviour:

B6.1 Placating

Step on a *placator's* foot and they will be the one to apologise. Placators know that peacemakers get blessed – or at least don't get trashed. And so a typical placator will soothe, please and pacify those with whom they come into conflict.

More females than males tend to be placators. They tend to dislike disagreeing with people – even if they are being criticized.

The aim of the placator is to get others to be nice to them – and, as placators tend to be externally influenced, they'll therefore probably go along with whatever the other person wants. They'll hold eye contact, smile a lot, and nonverbally ask for forgiveness. They apologize a lot, which means they tend to overdo it.

This type of behaviour prevents you asserting your rights; asking for what you want; and communicating how you feel. Protracted use of this approach may also tip over into retaliatory aggression when you've collected enough brown stamps to warrant a big bust-up!

To apologize a lot *from a position of weakness* – (suggesting that 'I'm Not OK') is bad for your sense of self-esteem. But to apologize reasonably frequently, *from a position of* **strength** – suggesting that 'I'm OK, and so are you' - for *accidental* and *unintended* negative impacts upon others, is **not** bad for your sense of self-esteem, and could be good for your relationships.

~~~

B6.2 Blaming

If a **blamer** steps on someone's foot, they will expect the other person (whose foot they stepped on) to apologize. This is because a blamer's classic move is to shift the responsibility away from themselves.

There are many ways in which they can do this: They can nag; they can sulk; they can shout; and they can hit out. Or they can pretend that it's not a problem and then launch a surprise attack a few hours later when everyone thinks the worst is over. This type is linked to the core of anger and aggression. While aggressive people blame and criticize; assertive individuals make *reasonable complaints* about *particular behaviours* (without damning the other person).

~~~

B6.3 Distracting

Did they step on someone's foot? No! A **distracter** will state that they weren't even there. They'll smile, or crack a joke, or say what lovely weather it is today, and do everything they can to deflect attention from the issue at hand. Their favourite phrase is this: 'It wasn't me'. This is manipulation, and can be linked to indirect aggression.

~~~

B6.4 Computing

When a *'computer'* steps on someone's foot, they simply won't register the fact. They are the one who just doesn't seem to feel anything, and they don't respond emotionally to what's happened. They simply shut down their feelings – and can't understand the suffering of others, if it is (or seems to be) illogical or irrational. Or just plain 'emotional'! (They may seem somewhat autistic, or alexithymic [not understanding feelings], or emotionally unintelligent).

When a *computer style* is used by a person, it may seem like they are simply responding calmly to a crisis. But they are panicking just as much as anyone else. It's just that they are trying to handle their panic by cutting themselves off at the neck. And actually, that's just as bad an idea as placating, blaming or distracting, because they are missing out on the information or motivation their body is trying to give them.

So they will take action, but over-rationally. And they will respond, but insensitively. (This is a common side-effect of studying 'rational therapy' and some forms of CBT!)

~~~

B6.5 Levelling

The final personal conflict style is the only healthy one: *Levelling*, or straight communication!

A *leveller* who steps on someone's foot will notice. Then they'll move back, and apologize appropriately. Then they'll ask if there's anything they can do. They won't grovel, dump the information, or look the other way – and they won't cut off from their feelings. They'll be genuinely regretful – but unlike people who run the other four personality sub-patterns, they won't go into a spiral of defensive responses.

So *a leveller* is going to be the one to hang in there under stress or in conflict, and simply get things sorted out. They will strike a balance between thinking and feeling – and that means that they will:

(a) Face up logically to the problem; and:

(b) Have the emotional energy to sort it out.

Whether at home or in the wider world, they'll have the space to listen to other people, take into account everyone's needs, and find a solution. And they will also assert their own needs in a reasonable manner.

Anyone who works with a leveller, marries a leveller, or has a leveller for a friend, therefore has an easy life. They know exactly where they stand with a leveller, and consequently feel secure. They know that if any problems arise in their relationship, then the leveller will tell them. (They will not whine, sulk, push the problem away or deny their feelings).

The bottom line is that the more positive your upbringing, and the more assertive your parents were, the more likely you are to be a leveller. (If you were not raised in this way, you could still be a leveller, if you had some corrective experiences, in social relationships or therapy, or assertiveness training, later in life).

~~~

B6.6 Learning to level

It might now be obvious that the first four 'types' listed above could benefit from learning how to level with others: or to speak up and describe what is happening, and how they experience it.

Being a heavy-duty *placator, blamer, distracter,* or *computer,* isn't a particularly good idea. Not only do these personality sub-patterns feel uncomfortable to use in practice, but they also will not be appreciated by your partner, your work colleagues, or by your friends and family.

Of course, everyone runs a bit of the four unhelpful personality sub-patterns, at least some of the time. This is not surprising, because, when we are young, in our family of origin, we learn ways of behaving that *seem* to work; or that seem to be normal. And at school, skills at maths and English and other subjects are rated much more highly than the ability to deal with people effectively and skilfully.

IQ (or the ability to take logic tests) is rated much higher than EQ (or the ability to read one's own emotions; the emotions of others; and to communicate about both). But when we grow to adulthood, the limitations of our lack of skill in handling conflict do begin to become much clearer. Virginia Satir's therapeutic advice was to shift your behaviour towards *helpful 'levelling'.*

B6.7 Some tips on the various styles

The limitations of the different ways of handling conflict will now be outlined:

1. If you tend to be a placator:

    (a) You may think it's a good sub-pattern as it seems to smooth things over.

    (b) However, you won't get what you want. And you can drive people crazy by always apologising.

    (c) To move towards being a leveller, you have to learn to have strong personal boundaries; and higher self-esteem; and to know how to communicate assertively.

    ~~~

2. If you tend to be a blamer:

    (a) You may think it's a good sub-pattern because at least no one shouts at you.

    (b) In fact, it alienates people. And, by shifting responsibility, you give away your power.

    (c) On the other hand, to move towards being a leveller, you have to realize that the world is not out to get you; and that temper tantrums don't work. You need to move back from aggression towards more reasonable self-assertion.

    ~~~

3. If you tend to be a distracter:

    (a) You may think it's a good sub-pattern because it gets you off the hook or out of the soup.

    (b) In fact, you never get to face problems. And you never take responsibility for things. (And taking responsibility is the first step towards solving most of your problems!)

    (c) Instead, to move towards being a leveller, learn to face up to it when other people challenge you. Then either take their criticisms on board, or stand firm in believing their criticisms are invalid. Face the truth!

~~~

4. If you tend to be a computer:

(a) You may think this is a good way to behave, because it keeps you clear of 'messy emotions'.

(b) In fact, you miss out by ignoring your own feelings and the feelings of significant others. And you may come across as hard-hearted, or cool, or cold and detached. If you cannot read another person's emotions, then you cannot really understand them or communicate effectively with them.

(c) To move towards being a leveller, allow yourself to pay more attention to what you are feeling, and what those feelings tell you about the value of what is happening to you. Allow yourself to pay attention to what other people are feeling; and take their emotions into account. (You might need some coaching in the labelling of emotions; and understanding how to manage them in yourself. [See Appendix E: Understanding and managing human emotions]). Try to grow your emotional intelligence.

~~~

One of the primary aims of being a leveller is to preserve feelings of self-worth all round; and to protect the dignity all the participants in communication with each other. According to Virginia Satir:

"Feelings of worth can flourish only in an atmosphere where individual differences are appreciated, mistakes are tolerated, communication is open, and rules are flexible - the kind of atmosphere that is found in a nurturing family".

Satir's approach is also designed to promote 'the five freedoms', which are defined like this:

1. To see and hear what is here, now; and not what should have been here; what was (previously) here; or what may be here in the future.

2. To say what one thinks and feels, instead of feeling constrained by unreasonable rules imposed by others.

3. To feel what one actually feels, instead of working to substitute 'racket feelings' imposed by others in the past.

4. To ask for what one wants, instead of passively waiting for permission from others to do what they want you to want.

5. To take calculated risks on your own behalf, instead of choosing to play it ultra-safe in a tiny 'comfort zone'.

B7 Conclusion: Learning new behaviours

As you can see from the description above, the behaviour of someone who is a 'leveller' is the ideal style of communication that we can work towards, if we want to work well with other people, and have a healthy, loving relationship with a significant love-partner.

But it isn't easy! You have to put in some considerable effort to bring about personal change.

We never stop learning how to deal with people. The quiz and descriptions shown above should help you to know the strengths and weaknesses of your personal style. And this document makes the case for moving towards being a leveller, and provides some guidelines for doing so.

The 'levelling' approach;

> - reduces conflict (in the long-term, and overall; though the best relationships exist on the other side of conflict [provided the conflict is based on 'fair fighting']). It also

> - reduces stress in our bodies, because we are dealing with problems *as they arise,* by facing up to them.

The reality is that we can't change other people – only ourselves! (And that, as you most likely know already, is not easy – but it's often possible, with enough effort and commitment to change!)

By moving increasingly towards being a leveller, we can earn our own self-respect - (which as Lord Roseberry said, is worth fourteen times more than the approval of other people) - and we can become a really good role model for our children (if we have them) and other people in our environment.

Virginia Satir's model helps us to see where we are operating from; and also what works and what doesn't, when it comes to dealing with conflict constructively.

When you level with another person, you may feel nervous. And 'the boat' of your relationship may *rock* for a little while - (a few minutes to a few hours).

But this rocky period will pass; and in the process you will be moving through the conflict, and out the other side: which is the gateway to better relationships. Because, as Robert Bolton (1979) writes:

"The best relationships exist on the other side of conflict"!

You cannot get there if you resist conflict – or if you resist levelling with your partner!

~~~

Copyright (c) Renata Taylor-Byrne, Hebden Bridge, November 2018.

~~~

Appendix C: Self-Assertion

C1: Introduction

Most people do not know how to communicate *assertively*. Communicating assertively means: asking for what you want; and saying 'no' to what you do not want; while at the same time showing respect for your own rights and the rights and sensibilities of the other person.

Some people are *too passive*, and behave like door-mats to their partners.

And some are *too aggressive*, and 'go to war' with their partner at the drop of a hat!

Here's a really surprising insight, from Professor Howard Markman, who is the Director of the Centre for Marital and Family Studies at the University of Denver, Colorado:

"When women bring up issues, men tend to withdraw because *they are afraid of fighting*. We (at our centre) train men to *listen* to what their wife is saying, instead of closing down". (From Agnew, 1996).

(See Chapter 4, of my book on couple relationships (2018)[148], for our introduction to effective communication strategies – including active listening, and formal listening time).

A similar point was made by Professor John Gottman, at the Gottman Institute in Seattle, Washington. In his main book on marriage, Gottman (1997) writes that, in 70% of cases of volatile conflict between couples, it is the man (not the woman!) who fills up with stress hormones, and then closes down, because he cannot think while his brain is awash with adrenaline. (See also: Kiecolt-Glaser and colleagues, 1996)[149].

So more women than men are aggressive in their communication, and more men than women withdraw - (according to Kiecolt-Glaser, [1996]; Gottman [1997]; and Markman, in Agnew's [1996] newspaper article.).

Many women make the mistake of thinking men are so tough that they can be spoken to in any old rough manner at all, and they should be able to handle that kind of approach! But, in most cases (perhaps 70% of conflicts), *they can't!*

This is how Agnew (1996) expresses Professor Markman's view:

"Women ... (in Markman's relationship program) are encouraged to request a time to discuss a problem, rather than (a classic female error, apparently) demanding to have it out the moment the man walks through the door. ... What both sexes need ... is understanding rather than agreement".

~~~

However, there are many situations in which women feel *too vulnerable* to speak up, in case their partner becomes verbally or physically aggressive. This has been researched by a group of scientists in Maryland, US, and reported by Dr Elaine Eaker in 2007. It turns out that women who 'bite their tongues' during rows are four times more likely to die earlier than those who shout back. But this probably applies no matter what your gender happens to be, and the researchers conclude that "Both spouses really need to allow another person a safe environment to express feelings when they're in conflict".

~~~

Whether a couple have a relationship riven by conflict; or one in which they fail to communicate about their feelings; or one where one partner plays aggressive Top Dog while the other plays passive Under Dog – they are likely to be living in misery, and also making each other physically and mentally sick. (See Umberson, et al., 2006). Here is an extract from the abstract of Umberson's report:

"...marital strain accelerates the typical decline in self-rated health that occurs over time and ... this adverse effect is greater at older ages. These findings fit with recent theoretical work on cumulative adversity in that *marital strain seems to have a cumulative effect on health over time* – an effect that produces increasing vulnerability to marital strain with age. Contrary to expectations, *marital quality seems to affect the health of men and women in similar ways across the life course.*"

New research at Ohio State University, in 2018, led by Dr Janice Kiecolt-Glaser, shows how conflicted marriages make people physically unwell. "We think that this everyday marital distress – for some people – is causing changes in the gut that lead to inflammation and, potentially, illness".

(Kiecolt-Glaser, quoted in Knapton, 2018. See also, Kiecolt-Glaser, Wilson and Bailey, et al., (2018) and Ohio State University (2018))[150].

And we already know that leaky gut can trigger leaky blood-brain barrier, resulting in toxins getting into the brain, and affecting moods and emotions. (Enders, 2015: Pages 114-133).

So, nobody escapes. Marital strain and conflict affects men and women about equally; and this effect is likely to harm both *physical health* and *emotional wellbeing.*

And my proposed solution is that the partners in conflicted marriages - to avoid bad-tempered fights - should learn how to *communicate* more effectively; to have *personal boundaries*; and to know how to *assert their legitimate rights.*

~~~

In this chapter I have set out to introduce you to the most basic level of self-assertion skills.

This is because it can be profoundly demotivating to be introduced to skills which are just too difficult – or 'too scary'! – to be implemented.

So, instead, I am going to teach you a range of knowledge and skills which can fairly easily be implemented by almost any reader of this book.

If you have any difficulty implementing any of the ideas in this chapter, you could discuss how to proceed with a good coach, counsellor or psychotherapist, who can guide you through any difficulties that you experience.

However, my expectation is that, in most cases, you will find this material easy to work with, and experience no significant difficulty applying the knowledge and skills described below.

C2: Passivity, assertion and aggression

If you want to be clear about the distinction between passivity, assertion and aggression, as forms of human behaviour, then the best model to use is this:

All human behaviour can be mapped on a continuum from passive to aggressive, via assertive; as shown in Table B1 below.

Passive	Assertive	Aggressive
Passive behaviour involves putting up with aggressive or bullying behaviour by others. Failing to ask for what you want. Giving in to others and being overly-compliant. Using flowery and diplomatic language to placate others. And being unwillingness to pursue your own needs and interests.	Asking for what you want. Saying no to what you do not want. Negotiating fairly about differences of opinion or clashes of interests. Owning your own viewpoint, by stating that "I wish..."; "I want..."; "I would like..."; etc. Rather than 'You-Statements' (like those in the *Aggressive* column). Expressing appreciation for what is given; expressing *conditional appreciation* for what is requested.	Aggressive behaviour involves treating others unfairly, by intimidating them, or demanding that they comply with your wishes. Aggressors offend against others in pursuit of their own interests. This often involves anger and verbal hostility. Can include physical violence. Blames others and fails to take any responsibility for their own actions. Points finger of blame, and over-uses You-Statements: "You should..."; "You must..."; "You have to..."; etc.

Table C1: Some indicators of passive, aggressive and assertive behaviour

Putting up with unfair treatment by one's partner is not a good way to build a happy sex-love relationship (nor any other kind of relationship), since the conformity and compliance will build up into resentment of the dominator. It is much better for both parties to the relationship, and for the relationship as an institution, for both partners to behave in an assertive way with each other. This book will help you to learn how to do just that.

One of the problems that was identified by Gestalt Therapy theorists is that many couples tend to play an unhealthy psychological 'game', called Top-Dog/Under-Dog.

I have dealt with many couples where this game was played on a win-lose basis from week to week.

At the first session of couple's therapy, the couple would come in, and one of them would be 'inflated' (or 'puffed up') and the other would be 'deflated' (or depressed).

Before the second session, I would anticipate how that new session might go, but my guesses would be wrong, because this time the *previously deflated partner* would be *puffed up*, and the previous 'Top-dog' would now be the 'Under-dog'!

It was a *war* in the name of relationship! A sick game of "I'm the King (or Queen) of the castle. Get down you Dirty Rascal!"

If this is the kind of relationship (or, rather, 'involvement') that you have – or some variation on the gender war (or the partner war, in the case of gay relationships) – then the solution is to adopt the position, in principle, of Equal Dog – Equal Dog.

Refuse to entertain the idea that your partner could ever be *reduced in status or worth* in your relationship. **Insist** upon total equality for the two of you – no exception; no debate!

Make a commitment to end the war. **Commit** to total equality. **Commit** to fair (assertive) fighting about *interests*, and not *positions*. **Commit** to assertive communication; win-win encounters; and Equal Dog to Equal Dog relationship.

C3: Realistic and reasonable assertion

"'It is very important for couples to be able to express negative feelings, and it's normal to disagree. It's how you handle the conflict that predicts your future', says Professor Markman". (Agnew, 1996).

What is *legitimate assertion* of your wants and needs, and what is *excessive aggression* in pursuit of a win-lose strategy of relating?

Table C1 above contains the briefest of answers, which I will elaborate here:

C3.1. Asking for what you want

Asking for what you want is legitimate self-assertion. But bear in mind that you will not always get what you ask for. Why not? Because if it is legitimate for you to influence your partner into giving you what you want, then, according to the Golden Rule, it is also legitimate for your partner to influence you into giving them what they want. How can this be resolved?

Once you have committed to formal equality in your relationship, there is only one way to resolve this apparent tension, and that is to agree that each partner is entitled to influence their partner up to, but not beyond, *50% of the influencing* that is done over time.

Of course, it is not perfectly easy to measure how much your partner has influenced you, and how much they have reciprocated when you wanted to influence them. So some *goodwill* is needed. And a *cool* head. And a *warm* heart. And *an abandonment of petty squabbling* about crumbs that fall when the biscuit (or cookie) is broken in virtually equal halves!

When you want to ask your partner for something, make sure you have previously used 'appreciation messages' (or messages of thanks) – as described below, in section C3.5. Then use a '*conditional* appreciation message' – like "I would really appreciate it if you would agree to (X)". (See section C3.6 below).

C3.2. Saying no to what you do not want

Saying 'No' is legitimate assertion. Unless, that is, your saying 'No' shows up for a jury of your peers as *an intransigent refusal* to allow your partner to influence you to the same degree (on average) to which you try to influence your partner.

Of course, we all have red lines. And our partners should not expect us to cross any of our own red lines. However, if you have so many red lines that it is virtually impossible for your partner to influence you anywhere near as much as you influence them, then they will almost certainly conclude that you are *not really committed to equality* in the relationship – and that will begin to pull the relationship apart! So, if you want to keep the relationship happy, durable, peaceful and secure, then you have to try to meet your partner halfway, as much as is humanly possible.

Opt for the middle way between saying 'No' too often, and saying 'No' too infrequently. When your partner asks you for something, and you feel a resistance, ask for time to think it over. Take the time, and check out your feelings. Is this a reasonable request? Is it unreasonable in any way? Do you 'owe it' to your partner to let them influence you this time, because they have let you influence them on sufficient occasions in the past? Does this request breach any of your 'red lines'? Is it immoral; or illegal; or would it cause you physical pain or emotional distress? If, on balance, you want to say no, then resolve to do so! And stick to your refusal, if it is a matter of principle!

Teach yourself that it's okay to say 'No'. If you do not have the right to say 'No', then you have no personal boundaries: no personal power. So own that power; and clarify those boundaries. You can practice saying 'No' in role plays, with a friend. Ask your friend to pretend they are having a party on Saturday night, and they want you to come. Their job is to think of at least seven sentences of invitation, including inducements. For examples:

Friend: "I'm having a party on Saturday night. Would you like to come?" (1).

You: "No!"

Friend: "I can lay on your favourite food. What is your favourite food?" (2a)

You: "Chinese" (for example).

Friend: "I'll lay on some wonderful Chinese food. Say you'll come to my party". (2b)

"No!"

Friend: "What's your favourite music?" (3a)

Etcetera, etcetera.

Your friend keeps trying to put pressure on you to attend the party, and you keep saying "No!"

And keep your face straight. Do not try to soft soap them with a smile. Do not let your posture droop. Stand up straight, and tell it how it is. "No! I don't want to come!"

After about six or seven attempts to persuade you, the most persistent person will normally give up and accept your refusal as being okay!

C3.3. Negotiating fairly

Here is another example of reasonable assertion: Negotiating fairly about differences of opinion or about clashes of interests. And negotiating fairly means: (1) separate the people from the problem; (2) put the problem on the table and stand side by side to address it; (3) the problem is the problem – and your partner is not the problem; (4) talk in terms of your interests and not your positions; (5) seek to find out what is 'underneath' each of your interests; (6) seek to find some way of trade off on the basis of what is underneath your interests.

C3.4. 'Owning your own viewpoint'

This is another expression of reasonable self-assertion. 'Owning your own viewpoint' involves admitting that "This is how it looks to me!"; rather than "This is how it IS!!!"

Instead of insisting that "It has to be like this...", consider using some preferential statements like these: "I wish..."; "I want..."; "I would like..."; etc.

This is much more democratic and fair than making absolutistic 'You-Statements', like these: "You should..."; "You must..."; "You are wrong, and I am right about...", etc.

Another important way of looking at this issue is to note that, in Transactional Analysis – (which is explored in Appendix B of Byrne, 2018b) – there is a distinction made between 'Parent language' and 'Adult language'.

Adult language involves the use of 'I-Statements': "I wish..."; "I want..."; "I would like..."; etc.

Parent language, (and especially Controlling Parent, and Critical Parent), is based on 'You-Statements'; for examples: "You should..."; "You must..."; "You have to..."; "You are wrong, and I am right about...", etc.

Another way of saying the same things is this:

Adult language normally consists of making *preferential* statements: "I would *prefer it* if you would... (do X instead of Y, [for example])". An exception would be when it comes to *defending your boundaries*, in which case you would use **a stronger I-statement**, like this: "I am *unhappy* about that behaviour, and I **will not** go along with...(X)".

C3.5. Expressing appreciation

Thanking your partner for what is given to you by them, or done by them, for you, or for your joint home life, is another form of assertive behaviour. "Thanks for .... I really appreciate it that you ... (did X)" "I like the fact that you (did Y) which allowed me to (do Z)..." "Thanks for that nice cup of tea (or walk in the country; or kiss on the cheek!)"

Thanking your partner for the things they do or say - which have a positive effect upon you - is important. The reason that it's so important is described by Helen Clinard (1987).

She calls this the skill of 'tracking positives'. She explains that it builds the self-esteem and the self-confidence of the person whose actions are appreciated. (And that's good for the health of the relationship!)

But she also points out that we each have a responsibility to teach our social environment - (which means the people around us, including our sex-love partner) - what we like and what we do not like.

The *appreciation message* helps us to teach them what we like.

C3.6. Using conditional appreciation messages

These differ from *appreciation* messages, in that *appreciation messages* are about the **previous** actions or words of your partner, while *conditional appreciation* is about the preferred *future* actions or words of your partner.

Let's take a look at an example:

Let us assume I want to walk in the park, because it's a nice, sunny afternoon, and I'd like my partner to go with me. I could say:

"I'd *really appreciate it* if you would join me for a walk in the park".

My partner has three (main) options:

1. She could *agree* to go with me; on the basis that I have often done things that she requested of me;

2. She could point out that this is a *bad time* for her, and suggest an alternative time which would work for her. (This might reflect a boundary she has, like this: "I must get my daily quota of writing done before I go out to 'play'!" And if that is her boundary, I would want to honour it!)

3. She could attempt to negotiate a *different place* for our walk, and check to see if that would be *acceptable* to me as a compromise. (This might be based upon her *low threshold of boredom*; and the fact that I *often* want to walk around the park, while she likes more variety in her walking environments).

But the bottom line is this: I ask her *nicely,* in the context of *normally thanking her* when she does something nice for me; and this *combination* (of asking nicely, and thanking her as appropriate) enhances the chances of her agreeing to go with me. Or, to put it another way: Conditional appreciation messages tell your partner what you would like, and often what you would prefer them not to do, in the future (including the immediate future)! In this sense, conditional appreciation messages are a way to convey both my *desires* and my *boundaries* to my partner. And my boundaries are about "what I will allow in", and what I want to "keep out".

C3.7. The power of operating from the 'I'm OK - You're OK' position

Some marriage partners assume that they are "OK", meaning *good*; but that their partner is "Not-OK", or *a bad person*. These kinds of partnerships are based on a Boss and a Follower; or the *Top Dog / Under Dog* model.

In other relationships, those roles flip around. Sometimes the man is The Boss (or Top Dog), and sometimes the woman is the Boss (or Top Dog).

Sometimes the flip-around process is driven by what we call 'splitting'; a process in which Partner 'A' thinks their Partner (B) is Okay, so long as Partner 'B's behaviour is generally perceived to be good. But if Partner 'B' engages in some bad behaviour, then Partner 'A' perceives them as 'All Bad'. (See my description of 'splitting' in section 4.4 of Chapter 4 above).

We teach our couple clients to reject both inequality in their relationships (and playing 'Top Dog/ Underdog' is one example of a strong commitment to inequality). And we also teach them to give up 'splitting' their partner into Good and Bad, and to relate to them as a Whole-Imperfect being who sometimes does well, and sometimes under-performs. (This does not, however, including any *excuses for immorality*: like domestic violence, sexual abuse or sexual infidelity, and so on!)

One of the ways we get them to give up these forms of splitting and inequality is by teaching them *the OK-Corral model* from Transactional Analysis, which is shown in Figure C.1 below.

		Your Decision About Others	
		OK	Not-OK
Your Decision About Yourself	OK	1. I'm OK - You're OK	2. I'm OK - You're Not-OK
	Not-OK	3. I'm Not-OK - You're OK	4. I'm Not-OK - You're Not-OK

Figure C.1: The OK Corral for Transactional Analysis

This model helps people to understand that the healthy life-position to operate from is this: *"I'm OK and so are you (my partner)"* – just so long as we are both committed to acting as moral and socially-responsible individuals.

It also helps the individual to understand if they are operating from *negative attitudes* towards themselves or others. In TA, these could be classified as (conscious or non-conscious) *not-OK life-positions* (about self or others).

A *'not-OK' life position* could include either of the following attitudes:

(1) **"I'm not OK** because I cannot please my partner; (or I cannot get a job; or I cannot make a success of my career; or I cannot get along with others"; etc.) Or:

(2) **"You're not OK** because you frustrate me; (or threaten my self-concept; or because you challenge me in ways that make me feel uncomfortable)"; etc.

To have a happy couple relationship, you have to learn (or teach yourself) to always operate from the 'I'm OK – You're-OK' position, in your dealings with your partner. (The exception here is this: If your partner acts in a way which is clearly illegal or immoral – like using physical violence, or emotional bullying, or any form of coercion against you; or requiring you to do anything [for example, in the bedroom] which you really do not want to do, then they have crossed over into that territory which we call **'Bad Wolf'** **behaviour**, and you have to take action to stop them! [See Appendix F of Byrne 2018b]).

~~~

C4a: Use of assertive body language

Body language is non-verbal communication; or leakage of bodily signals about emotional states. For example, if you saw two individuals across the street, and somebody told you one of them had just been fired from their job (sacked, or made redundant), and the other one had just been promoted, would you expect to be able to see the difference, without asking them any questions? Of course you would. Even if your ability to read body language is not particularly conscious, and you could not describe how you do it, I am convinced you would look for differences between:

1. **The two faces**: Which one looks happier, perhaps smiling broadly; and which one looks most dejected, or sad, or neutral, or worried?

2. **The posture of the two bodies**: Which one is looking downwards, head bowed? And which one is looking upwards, or straight ahead? Which one has the straightest, most erect spine?

3. **Their pace of movement**: Which one looks most vigorous? Which one looks slowed down, or lethargic?

4. **Their use of eye contact**: Which one is making *more open eye contact*? Which one looks down or away the most?

5. **Body armouring**: Does one of them have their arms folded across their chest, in a form of 'body armouring', or self-protection?

I am quite confident you would know in a glance which one had been promoted and which one was sacked or made redundant.

And now, suppose you cross the street, and can hear not only what they are saying to each other, but also:

5. **Their tones of voice**: Which one sounds surer of themselves? Which one sounds less sure of themselves? Which one sounds happier? Which one sounds least happy?

Since you can easily read the body language and non-verbal communication of these two described individuals, you must realize that other people read your body language all the time. If you are to communicate your boundaries assertively, you have to take a close look at what messages you are sending to your partner non-verbally.

If there are any weaknesses in your boundaries, your partner (and others) will be able to pick them up, non-consciously, through your body language; and may often violate your boundary at those points, without thinking about the implications of such violations.

I teach my clients the importance of this aspect of self-assertion with the following story:

Back in the 1980's, when assertiveness training was popular in the UK and the US, a woman (Janet) went on a weekend assertiveness training workshop. She was very upset by a male colleague of hers (Stephen) who constantly messed her around in their shared office by:

1. Borrowing her staple machine, and not returning it; often mislaying it so she had to waste time hunting for it.

2. Removing files from her desk, and hiding them in his desk drawers, until she was so stressed out about the missing information that he could return the files to her while laughing, and demanding to know: "Can't you take a joke?"

3. Making jokes at her expense ("ribbing her"), and frustrating her and putting her down.

So, she went to the weekend workshop; she studied all the skills that they were teaching there; and spent her evenings planning how she would use those skills on Stephen to get him to stop giving her a hard time.

Then, on Monday morning she returned to work. In the foyer of her office building, she ran through the skills she's learned; and thought about which skill she's use when he did behaviour X, or Y, or Z. When she was psychologically prepared for the worst, she got into the lift (elevator), took three deep breaths; drew herself up to her full height and looked straight ahead at her image in the mirror; put on her best "Don't f*** with me" face; and pressed the button for the sixth floor.

The life whirred up to the sixth floor, Janet stepped out of the lift, crossed the hallway, pushed open the door, expecting immediate trouble from Stephen. Instead, what she saw was his jaw drop; his smile fade; and his eyes go down to the paperwork on his desk. She said *nothing*, went to her desk, and worked diligently all morning, until tea break, which she took with a colleague on the fifth floor. She returned to her desk and checked that her files and stationery items were all okay, and got on with her work. She went out for lunch with a friend; and returned to a quiet afternoon at her desk. At no point did she speak to Stephen. But he had got her *nonverbal message* loud and clear. "Do not f*** with me!"

Body language! Body language! Body language! (But if you have to state this boundary in language, remember to use *assertive* language, and not *aggressive* language).

~~~

C4b: What's wrong with passivity and aggression

If you are too *passive* and *compliant* in your relationships, then you are not going to get what you want from your relationships, and you may be oppressed or exploited, or neglected and abused. The **sad truth** of human relations is this; Bullies are **created** by victims at least as much as victims are created by bullies! So don't behave like a *victim*, or you will very likely become one!

On the other hand, if you are too aggressive and controlling in your relationships, you will alienate your partner, and destroy your relation-ships. If you are sceptical about this point, and think your partner should be able to handle your raising of your voice and expressing your frustrations in a volatile manner, then you need to know what the research by Dr John Gottman - one of the most respectable of marriage counselling researches – shows: One of Professor Gottman's most important research discoveries was this:

When one partner behaves in a volatile (or angry) manner, the other partner fills up with the stress hormone, cortisol, which effectively prevents them from being able to reason about what is going on; therefore they tend to withdraw.

This was true even in those cases where a small woman (wife) was volatile with a huge man (husband)!

For the two reasons stated above, what you need to be able to do is to find a 'middle way' between being *too passive* and *too aggressive*; and that pathway is called *'the assertive approach'*.

To find out just how assertive you are at the moment, please complete the Assertiveness Questionnaire shown in the next section.

C5: An assertiveness questionnaire

The more appropriately assertive you are, the less stress will you experience in your relationships. So, how assertive are you?

Here's a little quiz designed to allow you to find out.

Please tick column 1, 2 or 3 against each statement below.

A tick in column 1 means "Almost always".

A tick in column 2 means "Sometimes"

A tick in column 3 means "Almost never".

Assertiveness Questionnaire

Statements of assertive rights	Col.1: Almost always	Col.2: Sometimes	Col.3: Almost never
1. I believe I have a right to be treated with respect as an equal human being.			
2. I believe I have a right to ask for what I want, while recognizing that others have the right to refuse.			
3. I ask for what I want.			
4. I believe I have a right to make my own arrangements and agreements, without being controlled or bullied by others.			
5. I believe I have a right to change my mind, and to communicate that change.			
6. I believe I have the right to change my beliefs and behaviours.			
7. I believe I have a right to say 'No' to requests from others.			
8. In practice, I can and do say 'No' to unreasonable requests, or requests that I want to decline.			

...continued...

9. I believe I have the right to choose not to accept responsibility for others and their feelings and problems.			
10. I believe I have the right to say 'I don't know' or 'I don't understand'			
11. I believe I have the right to ask for more time or more information			
12. I believe I have the right to say 'yes' or 'no' and not feel guilty			
13. I believe I have the right to make mistakes and to take responsibility for them			
14. I believe I have the right to be independent of the goodwill of others (if I so choose) especially if the price of that goodwill is too high (as in unfair or unequal relationships).			
15. I believe I have the right to choose NOT to be assertive, when I want to choose that option			

C6: The mark scheme and the definition of assertiveness

To mark this questionnaire, please award yourself three points for each tick in column 1; one points for each tick in column 2; and zero points for each tick in column 3.

You are perfectly assertive if you scored 45 points (the maximum). You are totally passive if you scored zero points. And your level of assertiveness is most likely to be somewhere between those two extremes.

If you scored less than 30 points, then you need to do quite a bit of work to become optimally assertive.

Study the fifteen beliefs in this questionnaire, above, and try to move yourself towards a more consistent set of assertive beliefs and actions. This should reduce your stress level. It should also get your more of what you are legitimately entitled to ask for, without damaging your relationship with your partner.

By contrast, being *aggressive* is stress-inducing, in that, by definition it is a strong expression of the "fight response", and could produce an equally aggressive response from the victim of your aggression. You are already overly-aroused when you are angry. But it is doubly stressful because, immediately after an individual becomes aggressive, they are liable to become *fearful* that their victim might retaliate, so they then may tend to feel anxious, which is the other form of over-arousal, also known as the "flight response".[151]

Reasonable assertiveness is characterized by the following types of behaviour:

(1) **Asking** for what you want, instead of expecting others to read your mind;

(2) Saying **'No'** to what you do not want, in a clear and reasonable manner; and:

(3) **Communicating** your appreciation for the things provided by others. (Helen Hall Clinard, [1985][152]).

(4) Saying 'I **would** appreciate it…' - when you make a request;

(5) Telling your partner how their behaviour affects you: (Saying, "When you do (X), I feel (Y), because (Z)"). (Robert Bolton, 1979/1986). (This skill will be fully developed in Volume Two of this book series).

If you want to see, and study, some role models of *assertive behaviour*, then you could go to YouTube, and search for videos on the following subjects:

"Saying No assertively"; "Asking for what you want"; or "Assertive communication".

~~~

C7: Postscript on assertiveness skills

Assertiveness is the form of moderate-anger-expression to aim for, because it is respectful of both parties to a conflict, and it minimises damage to the relationship and to the health and self-respect of the asserting person: (Bolton, 1979; Clinard, 1985; Lindenfield, 2000[153]). Fisher (2005) presents a list of the main features of 'healthy anger, or 'assertiveness', and I have amended that list as follows:

(1)   Directness, openness, being up-front, honesty, clarity. This includes asking for what you want; saying no to what you consider to be unreasonable or unacceptable; and being willing to negotiate and compromise.

(2)   Honour, morality, principle, fairness, ethics, justice. This includes being clear about the justice or morality of your position; and treating the other person fairly.

(3)   Focus, concentration, engagement; which includes sticking to the relevant facts; avoiding overly emotional squabbling (or rhetoric); seriously examining ideas.

(4)   Persistence, constancy, determination; including: the use of repeating your requests ('broken record' technique); standing your ground; being true to your gut feelings and your ideas.

(5)   Courage, bravery, daring, guts, boldness, and audacity, intentionality: which includes, taking calculated risks; remaining calm and adult; being committed to both resolution and relationship.

(6)   Empathy, kindness, compassion, forgiveness, concern, consideration. This includes: being sensitive to the limitations of the other person, and not being judgemental; being able to listen to the other side of the argument; and being able to respect the humanity of the other party.

We should commit ourselves to communicating our anger in these assertive ways and to avoiding the following examples of aggressive anger (from Sloane, 2010, page 15)[154]:

° Threats – using aggressive words or tone of voice.

° Intimidation – which involves making the other person feel small and frightened.

° Destructive – of other people, their property, our own health, etc.

° Violent outbursts – such as punching objects, physically assaulting other people, at home, at work, or in public places.

° Being selfish – or refusing to think about anybody except yourself.

° Blaming others – refusing to accept responsibility, and passing the blame around.

° Acting in a grandiose manner – such as driving too fast, posturing, spending too much money, etc.

~~~

Study guidelines

Tick that you've read this Appendix once: ❏

Before you more on to Appendix D, please read this chapter again: ❏

And a third time: ❏

~~~

When reading and re-reading this chapter, please underline those points that seem most important to you.

Make notes in the margins, as necessary, as quick reminders of the content of a paragraph or a page.

And turn down the corner of the page, when the content is so important you want to find it again, quickly and easily.

~~~

Appendix D: Mike Fisher's anger management training; and how to 'complete' repressed emotional experiences

By Jim Byrne, copyright (c) Jim Byrne 2011-2019

~~~

D1: Introduction

Cognitive and Rational therapy tends to dismiss consideration of *stories from the past of their clients*, including angry clients.

They present this rationalization: Everything that happened to the client in the past is here in the present, so all we have to do is to deal with their *present thoughts and beliefs*, and we deal with the whole life of the client.

However, in this appendix, I want to demonstrate that this is far from being true. What gets overlooked is this: The client had *experiences* in the past, and those *experiences* either got narrativized or not. When a negative experience is **not** *narrativized* (or turned into a story) by a person, they most often get stuck with that experience, which rattles around in the basement of their mind, potentially causing emotional and behavioural problems in the present (and even physical illnesses).

It is only by revisiting those kinds of experiences in the past – which admittedly is not easy – and by *reframing* them, and *digesting* them, (normally in the form of *a new narrative*), that their negative charge can be drawn, and they can finally be filed away in an *inactive* file in long-term memory. (See Byrne, 2019)[155].

D2: A story of completion

In an article in the *Daily Mail Online*, (6th June 2011) [156], a student of Mike Fisher's[157] Anger Management training course – Philip Robinson, a journalist - wrote about his experience of participating in Mike's training.

According to the blurb about the article, Philip had struggled "to control his fury. Horrified at repeatedly raging at his children, he tried a very unconventional therapy run by anger expert Mike Fisher."[158]

This story is a very good illustration of the fact that, beyond the process of 'reframing experiences', and asserting yourself about anger-inducing problems, it may also be important to do something called 'completing your experience' of past events which you have probably repressed out of conscious awareness, and which now prime you for reactive angry responses, or rages, in the present moment. This involves 'digging up' past experiences which were not properly digested, and working them through to completion, or resolution.

Mike Fisher has designed an anger management training course, which lasts two days, which encourages participants to do just that: to dig up their past experiences, and to process them.

When events occur in our lives, we may:

(1) Note them, non-verbally, and be affected by them, emotionally, because they match some pattern from the past; or:

(2) We may note them, reflect upon them using words and ideas, digest them into the form of an intelligible story, and file them away.

Response (2) is what we call *'completing your experience'* of an event, while response (1) is called 'having an undigested, affective experience'.

To *complete* your experience of an event, you need to focus your attention on it, using language-based concepts, and try to make sense of it as part of the story of your life, or the story of you week, or day, or family, etc.

Being good at completing your experience of events in your life is called 'narrative competence'. Some people have good levels of narrative competence, and some have poor levels. This depends very much on how your parents processed their own experiences. If they operated with a 'restricted code'[159], they are unlikely to have had good narrative competence, and they will have been unable to teach you the 'elaborated code' which is essential for narrative competence.

When an individual has a particular kind of unpleasant experience, which they have not digested, it can tend to affect them in negative ways for the whole of the remainder of their lives, or until they dig it up and process it, complete their experience of it, and file it away in a satisfactory narrative format. (See Byrne, 2011)[160].

~~~

D3: An angry man completes his experiences from the past

Let me now present Philip Robinson's story, and I will comment upon it as necessary: Philip is in a constant state of angry scolding of his eight-year-old son. But no matter how much he scolds him, his son does not do what Philip is trying to intimidate him into doing. This clearly sounds like an **anger syndrome**, not just isolated instances of anger. And, you cannot *reframe the triggers* in the case of a syndrome (which you can in the case of isolated instances of anger-incitement).

Of course, it might work to begin to reframe each of Philip's 'noxious anger-inducing triggers', one after the other, but it might also be important to go a lot deeper, and look for something that has not been processed in the past.

Philip explains that his anger has induced him to smash computer printers, kicking holes in doors, dented walls, and thrown all manner of toys into the garden.

Albert Ellis, the creator of Rational Therapy (REBT), would say that Philip is behaving like a dictator. Or 'a big baby' – but would that help him to stop? Not necessarily, though it might help to some limited degree. General CBT would encourage Philip to do a cost-benefit analysis: *What does he gain, and what does he lose by his uncontrolled anger outbursts?* Again, how likely is that to help? In E-CENT, we would say that Philip has very poor 'affect regulation capability', which probably needs to be reprogrammed in a re-parenting *relationship*.

Meanwhile, Philip has no idea how to calm down, and he feels he is spiraling down into a worse place.

"It's not only me", he writes. "Recent statistics show the whole nation is getting angrier. The average Briton flies into a rage four times a day, and one in ten of us claims to have been in an accident caused by road rage".

The evidence is all around us. People are getting angrier, and some are going to prison, and some are going into hospitals.

"Recently", write Philip, "one Cardiff woman even smashed up her local bakery, causing hundreds of pounds worth of damage. The provocation? They'd sold out of her favourite cupcakes".

Much of this kind of anger may be down to greatly increased environmental stressors, and no improvement in the individual's ability to cope. Plus disrupted sleep, excessive use of junk food, lack of physical exercise, and alcohol abuse. There are ways of improving your coping strategies for dealing with stress, such as improved diet, daily physical exercise, meditation, etc. But most people are not aware of the need to increase their coping strategies.

Philip goes on to describe the enormous cost of anger problems to the health services; the increasing ubiquitousness of angry outbursts; and the way he spoils his family life by getting angry at his kids at the drop of a hat.

D4: The first day of training

So he signs up for Mike Fisher's anger management course; but on the way to the training centre, he is involved in a road rage incident, because he thinks the while van behind him is driving dangerously. (He writes that he "despises" this kind of behaviour, and refers to the driver as a "numbskull": two very good ways of making oneself angry!) So he slows down to *intentionally frustrate* the following driver, and hopes this driver will have some kind of stroke due to blood pressure, resulting from being so frustrated by his (Philip's) slow driving. (That is pretty sick!)

He goes on to write that he was five minutes late, due to his own slow driving; and that he was "bathed in a fury-induced sweat. I walk into the therapy room and find five equally blotchy, scowling men looking back at me. I take my seat knowing I'm in the right place".

Philip then describes the other course participants as: "...a 50-year-old Scotsman who argues with his daughter; a 38-year-old journalist (me) who screams at his son; a 43-year-old economist and product of a top boarding school whose temper is taking its toll on his marriage; a builder who flew into a rage because his wife bought a dress; a cantankerous Star Trek fan who hates the world; a jargon-spouting maths professor who claims (unconvincingly) he has nothing to be angry about; and a retired businessman who can't talk to his family without getting drunk and hostile".

They begin by discussing the things that trigger their anger. Then Mike explains his theory: "...we become angry when our needs are not met. Basic requirements include love, respect, the need to be heard - stuff without which it's almost impossible to succeed as a human being".

This is only partly true. We become angry when our needs are not met, and we frame that experience in a particular kind of way. Mike knows that. In his book, he explains that "Beneath our anger is the sense that our values, core beliefs (negative or positive) or goals are being threatened or invalidated in some way…" (Pages 54-55)[161].

When we are young, we particularly strong needs to be loved and cared for, and so not getting our needs met when we are young can have a more significant impact on our anger levels, at a time when we do not know how to manage our emotions any better. And if we do not know how to process that anger, it can stay around to cause problems in the ways we respond to frustrations later in life; even into advanced old age.

And if pain is inflicted upon us when we are young, we can use anger as a way to cover that up, instead of feeling it – processing it. (See Fisher, 2005, pages 66-67).

D5: We are born to love and be loved

Whether Albert Ellis likes it or not, we are born with the expectation that we will be loved; the innate desire to attach to a love object, which matures around the age of five to six months of age, when we form a definite preference for our own mother as our love object. (Up to that point, we are more accepting of various carers).

From that point onwards, when we do not get the kind of sensitive attention that we desire, we feel upset, and we can either express that upset, or hide it from ourselves. When we hide it from ourselves, we are storing up problems for the future.

But remember what I said earlier. We have certain rights, but do not make the mistake of *demanding* that our rights are met. As mature adults, we need to learn how to *negotiate* for what we want in life, and to be sensitive and caring with those people with whom we relate. Don't kick over the beehive if you want to collect honey. And, also as adults, we can learn that what goes around comes around. But it's not perfectly effortless to achieve those states. We may need therapy for an insecure attachment style; or we may be healed by a partner who has a secure attachment style, and who provides a secure base for us.

Philip then describes how Mike writes a long list of profound essentials on the board. Presumably, Mike wrote a list of basic human needs on the board, much like that which he presents in page 70-71 of his book. This is a secondary consideration, after his view that people become angry when their values, beliefs and goals are thwarted invalidated. This is it:

"Some of the main primary needs are to be:

Valued	Safe	Significant	Cared for
Seen	Heard	Accepted	Appreciated
Acknowledged	Held	Touched	Respected
Encouraged	Useful	A member of the 'tribe' (belong)	Treated honestly
Treated fairly	Trusted	Loved	

Source: Fisher (2005), page 70-71.

Philip continues: "We head off into small groups to, as Mike says, 'shake the apple tree': identify incidents where we felt angry and pinpoint our unmet needs. No, I can't quite believe it either. My cynical side is straining at the leash".

And when I first read this statement, in 2011, I was also mystified: "Why are they going off to try to identify unmet needs?" I wondered; in those days I was much more influenced by the cognitive approach than I am today. So I wondered: "What about the more important and more fruitful area of *values, beliefs and goals?* Perhaps that will be dealt with later. Perhaps this first exercise is intended to bring up early childhood stuff and to deal with that first; and then to deal with later adult decisions about values, beliefs and goals".

However, I now recognize that there are *no conscious cogitations* that are *more important* than our earliest *emotionally-charged experiences*!

I (Jim) went on to think about it like this: "Another possible explanation is that Mike recognizes that it is not just the lack of some basic need that makes us angry, but also the way we frame it. However, since most of us with anger problems are likely to have framed them badly, in the past, and felt shame about looking at them, we may have repressed them into our 'shadow side', and now project them into our environment. We can use our current problems of anger to track back to see what needs are not being met, and then figure out how to meet them for ourselves.

Philip then describes some high risk conversations between the course participants, who have had no training in how to co-counsel; so this is a risky business, and ethically questionable. And it does end in upset emotions because one participant *makes another participant wrong*!

Philip continues: "We end the first day talking about 'the shadow': the memories, emotions and experiences deep inside us that, according to psychiatrist Carl Jung, control us unconsciously. The shadow is every issue in our past and present that we can't face: the events that shame us and make us feel worthless".

I (Jim) would like to clarify this a little: the Jungian theory says that we develop two aspects, or sub-personalities during our childhood development – the 'persona' and the 'shadow' side.

The persona is the socially shaped, and pro-social ego, or conscious 'personality';

And the shadow side contains all those manifestations of the 'bad wolf' that we have to repress out of awareness, because they make us feel guilty and ashamed, and threaten our survival as an accepted part of a social group (like family).

But it may also accidentally come to include some parts of us which are not objectively bad, but were felt to be unacceptable to our parents or society when we were young, such as excessive vitality, or flirtatiousness, or 'being different', or 'alien', or 'disappointing' to our parents. Thus we repressed them out of conscious awareness, and, as so often happens with repressed material, we tend to project our shadow side on to other individuals in our environment, and to attack it there.

Philip explains that the plan is to go home, and come back tomorrow to explore the contents of the shadow sides of each of the participants. He writes: "I go home exhausted, in time to kiss the family good-night. I don't feel hostile; I feel incredibly quiet".

Jim comments: Something has already changed for Philip. Perhaps just knowing the theory of the shadow has stopped him in his tracks. Perhaps something about the group processes in which people reveal those things that 'make them angry' has caused him to begin to 'get off it' about projecting his own stuff onto other people.

~~~

D6: The second day of training

The next morning, Philip is surprised to find that nobody has dropped out of the group, despite the difficult challenge they will face today.

Philip writes: "We seem more unified and calmer. The maths professor even apologies for being cold and shut off from the group. He says he thought about his behaviour all night and kept recalling an episode from his childhood when he was in hospital alone and terrified."

Wow (writes Jim). This guy has got in touch with repressed anxiety and fear about being in hospital all alone, and that has drawn the energy that used to fuel some of his anger!

"Mike explains we can all connect with him (the professor) now that he is being truthful, open and vulnerable. He tells us it's good to be like this, and if people want to reject that, you might ask yourself why you are hanging around them in the first place."

Don't hang out with people of low emotional intelligence, because they will feel obliged to drag you down to their own level.

Mike is encouraging the group members to be open about their thoughts and feelings, so they can be looked at, digested, processed, and filed away. This is very different from the more common approach of brushing our feelings under the carpet, where they fail to get processed, and they become part of our shadow, and get projected onto others, where we can safely attack them.

Philip continues: "I find myself agreeing. I feel dangerously close to quitting journalism and opening a pottery shop. The next step is the Detour Method. This is about looking at the big problem we walked in with and locating the event or issue behind it that's causing all the emotional distress and anger.

"Rory and I have a similar problem: we feel antagonistic towards our children when they disappoint us.

"I begin by identifying that I lose my mind and fly into a rage when Oscar doesn't do his schoolwork.

In Jungian analysis, unlike CBT/REBT, this Activating Event draws attention to something that has been repressed into the shadow side of the individual. The process of repression "…often leaves a psychic trace in our reactions to an assortment of different situations. These reactions often have no apparent logical explanation and are out of our control". (Fisher, 2005, page 76).

"Such reactions indicate that there is an ***underlying wound*** within us, and in order to heal this wound, we need to *explore these reactions* – preferably with the help of a therapist. Anything that is repressed controls us and will always return to haunt us – it's only a matter of time. Healing the wound means ***finding a way to come to terms with the dreadful memory we have repressed*** and (in the process) eliminating our inappropriate defensive thinking and responses towards others". (Page 76).

This process of "finding a way to come to terms with the dreadful memory we have repressed" is what I call "completing your experience" of undigested emotional events from the past. (Byrne, 2019).

Philip then describes how he begins to share something about himself, babbling, feeling clumsy, but suddenly "…the memory of screaming at my son unlocks a ball of anger, shame and embarrassment from my own childhood. I turn bright red and begin to stumble over my prepared script"

Another member of the group (Rory) asks him how old he was at that time, and he says 'ten'. And the incident that comes up from memory is a parallel of his own conflict with his son over doing his maths homework: "I'm at the dining room table with my Dad. It's Sunday afternoon and we're doing maths," and his dad is in a rage, just like he gets with his eight year old son, about maths homework.

This is what Freud called 'the compulsion to repeat' past experiences in our current life: shortened to the 'repetition compulsion'.

Rory is still prompting him with questions, and he responds: "My Dad is in a rage with me because I can't get the concept of vulgar fractions into my thick head. I want to leave, but he won't let me — not until I've got the question right. I stay, but I am too upset to learn anything, too stupid. I feel like a prisoner."

This is a perfect illustration of the process we have been describing above. Philip is shamed by his father, who treats him as if he is dumb, stupid, and Philip buys into that interpretation. But he cannot bear to incorporate the label 'dumb' into his persona – his conscious self-concept. And so he represses it into his unconscious shadow side; all those 'bits of himself' that hurt too much, or threaten to cause him too much anxiety or shame.

Years later, when he is a dad himself, he projects his repressed shadow side onto his own son, and attacks it there. He thus subjects his son to the same shaming experience he has hidden away from conscious awareness.

Rory then asks Philip what he (Philip) would say to his father, if they could go back in time, and Philip offers that he would ask his father why he wasn't nicer to him!

Rory tells him to make this statement louder, Philip does, and in the process he breaks down crying. He is back in touch with his childhood desire to be loved by his father, instead of being abused by him.

This is part of the process of 'completing the experience', which is necessary for healing, so that the traumatic experience can be digested and filed away in an 'inactive file'.

Philip continues his story like this: "I remember how scared I felt back then and how I could never speak up for myself. I realize how brave my son is: he dares to challenge me even though I'm 3ft taller than he is and much angrier than I remember my own father being. I have an overwhelming sense of revelation — and there is no animosity towards Dad. As a father myself, I understand why he did what he did; that he loved me and desperately wanted me to have every chance in life. I feel a rush of love for him, and my son, all at the same time."

In the process of *completing his experience* of that repressed event way back in his childhood, when he was ten, and could not do his maths homework, he somehow gets that his father was not his enemy – his father loved him. And he also gets that he loves his own son, who is brave enough to stand up to him. Undigested emotional experiences are getting processed and filed away into 'inactive files' where they will no longer cause any problems of emotional activation, projected out into the world.

This is a real Eureka moment for Philip. He realizes that he can (and will) be a better parent. He is moving towards a commitment to be kinder to himself, and to his wife and sons.

'Bloody hell!' says Rory, wiping away his own tears. 'I bet you didn't expect that.'

These are the tears of catharsis, of completion, of letting go of the past so it can be laid to rest at last.

~~~

D7: Philip's emotional transformation

Philip drives home with a calm and peaceful mind. The big bully who used to dominate his inner dialogue, has gone: kicked out as no longer needed or wanted or liked.

Philip continues his story: "At home, I talk to my little Oscar. He tells me how I wasn't nice to him. As he talks, he starts to cry. And then I cry, and I'm able to tell him that Grandad used to argue with me in the same way when I was little. I tell him I'm sorry I got angry, but that I love him a lot".

This is a lovely example of honesty about emotions, of getting them out in the open, talking about them, processing them, and allowing them to be filed away.

The conversation ends with Oscar and Philip realizing that this period of their life is over, and they hug each other lovingly.

Philip continues: "It's two weeks since the anger therapy finished and I can't quite believe how much it has changed my life. I feel in control. I don't get angry like I used to. When I feel the rage boiling up inside me, instead of screaming and shouting, I try to use it as an opportunity to look into my past and find out what I'm really upset about."

This is an example of a person using a disturbing event to check on the contents of *their shadow* (or aspect of the *repressed past*) which might otherwise be projected onto somebody else, instead of being made conscious and processed.

Philip ends his story like this: "Even the children are getting used to talking out their anger and frustration, as I now do. Our house feels warmer, calmer and more positive. If all this continues, I might be happy for my children to turn out like me after all".

~~~

Source:

Robinson, P. (2011) 'Could I send Mr. Angry packing?' An article in the 'Femail' section of the *Daily Mail Online*. 28th April 2011.

~~~

D8: Observations and comments by Jim Byrne

Appropriate anger which comes from the persona, or the socialized individual personality, is normally healthy and helpful, and normally expresses itself as *self-assertion*.

Excessive anger which is out of proportion to the actual situation may be coming from the shadow side, which has been repressed and then projected into the social environment. Or as Mike Fisher says:

"…we need to ask ourselves,

*(X): 'What part of my shadow is this person mirroring for me now?' (This question is **marked X** by Jim, for later reference back).

What does that mean? It means that, for example, if I repress my self-hatred, I am likely to project it onto others as them being hateful towards me. But are they really being hateful towards me, or am I misinterpreting their attitude because of my own buried self-hatred?

If I imagine they are being hateful towards me, I may respond with inappropriate anger or rage.

However: "The more you ask yourself this question", (marked X, above, by Jim) writes Fisher, "the more of your shadows you will uncover, and the more shadows you uncover – and, more importantly, befriend – the freer you will be of reactive anger…" (Page 76).

It is therefore obvious that we should use angry outbursts of an inexplicable or reactive nature to track back through our personal histories, and to try to find which bit of our own emotional experience we could not handle at that time. Which bit did we feel we had to repress out of conscious awareness. Now is the time to dig it up, look it in the eyes, and face up to the denied pain of that experience: the shame, guilt, anxiety, hurt, anger, or whatever; and chew through it, complete it, and allow it to be filed away in an inactive file.

If you cannot do this for yourself, then consider visiting a Jungian analyst (or an E-CENT counsellor) to get help.

~~~

Get your anger under reasonable control

Appendix E: Understanding and managing human emotions (with the emphasis on anger)

In this appendix I will present some substantial extracts from a previously published chapter on how to understand and manage human emotions – but I have deleted those sections that deal with anxiety and depression, and only left those that deal with anger.

This material was originally published as Chapter 7 of Byrne (2018a) Lifestyle Counselling[162].

~~~

E1: Introduction

Because counsellors and psychotherapists deal with their clients' *emotions* - (as well as their behaviours, goals, relationships; plus their environmental stressors, and so on) – every system of counselling and therapy has to have *a theory of emotion*. This, however, is a significant problem, for three reasons:

1. **Firstly**: Human emotion is hugely complex. For example, Stephen Pinker, in his book on how the mind works, draws attention to a quotation from G.K. Chesterton about the *unutterable complexity* of human emotional tones and moods and shades, which begins like this:

"Man knows that there are in the soul tints more bewildering, more numberless, and more nameless than the colours of an autumn forest". (Page 367)[163].

Therefore, at the very least, we should show some humility in developing our systemic models of such complexity.

2. **Secondly**: As one psychotherapist has pointed out:

"The terms 'feeling' and 'emotion', and 'affect' are used in many different senses in psychology. A review of more than twenty theories of emotion reveals a plethora of widely diverging technical definitions. These vary with the technique of investigation, the general theoretical framework, and the value-judgements of the psychologist. Often, they are so diverse as to defy comparison let alone synthesis".[164]

So we are not going to arrive at a universal definition of emotion in this book; though we have to come to some working hypotheses, in the form of practical conclusions, which allow us to understand and help our clients.

3. **Third**: There is a good deal of confusion regarding whether emotions are innate, or socially imposed; and whether they exist 'inside the client' or 'outside' in social relationships.

With regard to point 3, which is the most fundamental question we face, we should resolve that issue up front:

In E-CENT counselling, we use the insight from Dylan Evans' (2003) book on emotion, about 'degrees of innateness or learned emotions'. This means that we accept the conclusion that some basic emotional wiring is innate, at birth. However, those basic emotions (or feelings, or affects) are inevitably shaped by the culture of the mother (and father [normally]) into *acceptable* and *unacceptable* expressions of affect – or observable manifestations of feelings - over time. The main concepts we use are:

(1) Innate emotional wiring (Panksepp 1998) like, anger, fear, disgust, sadness, etc.; which are also seen as basic emotions[165] – (Siegel, 2015);

(2) Higher cognitive emotions (like pride, confidence, guilt and shame, jealous, trust and so on – (as in Panksepp and Biven, 2012); and:

(3) Culturally specific emotions: (For example: the ways in which various universal emotions are **manifested** *differently* in different cultures; e.g. the more restrained Japanese versus the more expressive Americans – (Evans, 2003).

Somewhere between the universal, higher cognitive emotions and the culturally specific emotions, I would place the "family variations" in the range and mode of expression of the basic emotions and higher cognitive emotions.

So, individuals have some of the 'universal shape' implied by Plato, Freud, Albert Ellis, Eric Berne, etc.; but also quite a lot of 'family shaping' which is idiosyncratic and unique. Plus national (and class) variations in how those emotions are expressed.

In evolving our theory of emotion, we went back as far as it is possible to go in developing knowledge of our ancestors, and what we inherited from them. For example, we have been influenced by the perspective of Jonathan

Turner (2000)[166], which can be summarized like this: "…our ability to use a wide array of emotions evolved long before spoken language and, in fact, constituted a preadaptation for the speech and culture that developed among later hominids. Long before humans could speak with words, they communicated through body language their emotional dispositions; and it is the neurological wiring of the brain for these emotional languages that represented the key evolutionary breakthrough for our species".

And according to Panksepp (1998), those emotional systems are located in the most primitive parts of the brain: the limbic system and brainstem. (These are the neuro-logical substrates (or foundations) underpinning what Freud called the 'It' – the *physical baby,* and the *primary (emotive) processes* of its mental life. Those primary, sub-cortical (limbic) processes inform our secondary, more culturally shaped emotions, which modulate our capacities for cognition: which means that our *attention, perception, memory,* and *thinking* can never be **separated** from our feelings. As Damasio (1994) demonstrated with his patient, Elliot, *we **cannot** make choices and decisions **without** the emotional capacity to **evaluate** options!* (We are *perfinkers,* (perceivers-feelers-thinkers) and not pure thinkers! [Glasersfeld, 1989]) .

Finally, in E-CENT counselling theory, we would never go along with a list of categories of emotional disturbances like that displayed in the *Diagnostic and Statistical Manual 5* (or any other *DSM*), or any other equivalent manual, such as the European's International Statistical Classification of Diseases.

Humans are too complex to be classified into 'disease boxes' or 'personality disorders'. And we will argue elsewhere in this book that much of the modern explosion of emotional disorders are a result of *lifestyle distortions,* especially in the areas of sleep deprivation, poor diet, lack of physical exercise, and rising levels of externally imposed socioeconomic stress. (See in particular, Appendix A, above).

~~~

Afterthought: However, despite the fact that we in E-CENT have clarified our own understanding of human emotions, there are lots of disagreements within the field of counselling and psychotherapy on this subject. Since there is no universal agreement regarding the nature of human emotions in counselling and therapy, we, in E-CENT counselling theory, have to account for our own theory of emotion: to justify it, as well as defining and elaborating its elements. So let us begin with some of the older theories of emotion.

E2: Buddhism and Stoicism on emotion

E-CENT counselling has been influenced by moderate Buddhist ideas and moderate Stoic ideas, including some of their ideas about human emotions. This is obvious from a reading of Chapter 3, on the Six Windows Model.

With regard to Buddhism, it seems from The Dhammapada[167], that the Buddha taught that all human disturbance arises out of *desire*; and this idea is shared with Stoicism.

In E-CENT theory we have taken some of these ideas as points of departure, but we have also found serious flaws in both of those philosophies.

For examples:

E2(a). Regarding Buddhist theory:

The opening lines of the Dhammapada are as follows:

"What we are today comes from *our **thoughts** of yesterday*, and our present thoughts build our life of tomorrow: *our life is the creation of our **mind***". (Page 1)[168].

In *my view*, it would be more accurate to say (or to *begin* by saying):

(1) "What we are today comes from *our thoughts (and **feelings**) **about our** experiences…*"

So, we are not talking about *disembodied thoughts*, devoid of a stimulus in an **external reality**.

And we are not talking about beings that can *think independently of their basic emotional wiring!*

People are emotionally wired up by their earliest relationships, and they live in the real world of good and bad experiences!

They have body-minds, and *their thoughts are strongly affected by diet, exercise, relationship support or its lack, external stressors*, and so on.

(2) "…and our present thoughts…" (*Plus our **feelings** and **actions**, including **eating**, **sleeping**, **relaxing**, **exercising**, etc.*) "…build our life of tomorrow…".

So our *thoughts* (about our *experiences*) **do not act alone**; they are not the **sole determinant** of our lives.

Let us then move on to the third element of the Buddha's statement:

(3) "…our life is the creation of our *mind*". E-CENT theory would suggest that that should be changed to this: Our life is the creation of our body-brain-mind-environment complexity. This includes the real world; *plus* our relationships; plus our experiences; plus our diet, sleep pattern, exercise; and our stressors – including economic and political circumstances, family life – and our coping resources - and on and on).

So the Buddha can easily *mislead the unwary*; as the unwary were misled by Albert Ellis and Aaron Beck – who both *downplayed* the role of the environment in human experience; with Ellis denying the role of early childhood in shaping the later life of the social-individual. Those theorists also overlooked the importance of our eating of unhealthy diets; and our failure to exercise our bodies; and our modern neglect of the importance of sleep; all of which impacts our emotional states.

To serve our clients well, counsellors and psychotherapists need to be *critical thinkers* (meaning *critical perfinkers!*); to be awake; to be well informed (meaning widely read, and subject to multiple influences); and to think (or perfink) for ourselves.

Buddhist ideology downplays the impact of the environment upon human organisms, in a way which is corrected by modern social psychology.

Social psychology is an attempt to understand and explain the various ways in which "we, as individuals are influenced by the actual, imagined or implied presence of others". Allport, (1985)[169].

If we are to develop a theory of human emotions, we must not follow the Buddhist dumping of this impact of the social environment on the thinking, feeling and behaviour of our clients, lest we end up **blaming the client** for their disturbance, as was done by Freud, Klein, Ellis and Beck. (Indeed, it was Dr John Bowlby who most strongly emphasized the importance of early childhood relational experiences: the impact, for better or worse, of our early social relationships upon our attachment style, and our chances of having a happy marriage in adult life. Because this went against both Freud's and Klein's perspective - [both of which blamed the child for their own emotional disturbances {which were assumed to result from phantasy!}] -

Dr John Bowlby was ostracized by the British psychoanalytic community for decades – because they insisted upon *blaming the clients' 'phantasies'* for their upset emotions.)[170]

~~~

However, the mindfulness aspect of Buddhism, especially Zen meditation, is very helpful for all of us, counsellors and clients alike, because it stops us ruminating on past problems, or anxiously anticipating future difficulties. Here is an illustration of how to understand 'mindfulness', or awareness of the present moment:

"The greatest support we can have is mindfulness, which means being totally present in each moment. If the mind remains centred, it cannot make up stories about the injustice of the world or one's friends, or about one's desires or sorrows. All these stories could fill many volumes, but when we are mindful such verbalizations stop. Being mindful means being fully absorbed with the momentary happening, whatever it is – standing or sitting or lying down, feeling pleasure or pain – and we maintain a non-judgemental awareness, a 'just knowing'." Ayya Khema[171].

However, here's one serious caveat: It is *not* a good idea to try to use mindfulness to suppress or deny our feelings about our distressing experiences. That will not work. We have to **file** our distressing experiences in the past, or they will **insert** themselves into our future! And the only way we know to file our distressing experiences in the past is to *experience their emotional content fully*; to *digest* those emotional experiences; to *complete* them; and thus to burn them up; and *file* them in inactive files in our long-term memory. This should also be combined with a re-framing process – like the Six Windows model – so that we get to *re-frame* old *traumatic experiences*; to see them differently; and to drain them of their original meaning.

~~~

E2(b). Regarding Stoic theory:

The most famous saying of the Stoic philosophers in the world of cognitive counselling systems today is this *extremist* belief:

"People are *not* upset by the things which happen to them, but rather by their *attitude* towards those things".

This *extremist* belief is central to Rational Therapy (REBT), and, though recent attempts have been made to shift to a conception of emotional upsets as being caused by the interaction of negative activating events and our beliefs about them, the basic instinct of REBT is to blame the client for holding 'irrational beliefs'. (Byrne, 2017).

Beck's Cognitive Therapy (CT) and CBT in general hold a more ambivalent attitude than REBT, with some emphasis given to the idea that "the event does not make you feel anything" - (Willson and Branch, 2006; page 12) – and the idea that it is only "sometimes" that the client "may assign extreme meanings to events", causing them to feel disturbed. (Willson and Branch, page 13). See also, Byrne 2017).

These extreme beliefs, of REBT, and certain aspects of harsh CBT, are also very similar to the opening statement of the *Dhammapada*, in that it both *blames the client* for their interpretation of their experience, and ascribes to them *the capacity to be indifferent* to their environmental insults, hurts and defeats. (This inference is clear from verses 2 and 3 of the Dhammapada, page 1). But only a lump of wood, or a stone, or some other inanimate object, can be truly indifferent to particularly intense environmental stimuli.

A *wise person* may well choose to ignore some environmental insults, hurts and defeats; to downplay them; or to *reframe them*, so they seem less painful. But not all of our clients can claim to be *wise* upon first encountering us. (And many of them will fail to achieve significant levels of wisdom; and almost none will rise to the level of Stoic functioning, just as most Stoics fail to rise to the level of the theoretical **'indifference to externals'** which Stoic theory demands of its adherents).

In time, we might teach some of our clients to be somewhat wiser - using some *moderate* Stoic principles – but we *should not* attempt to teach them the more extreme principles, such as that shown above; partly because we would have to *blame them* for their distress, to begin with; and then we would have to move on to *advocating super-human goals for mere humans.*

But there are some *moderate principles* of stoicism that we should try to practice and preach.

The most helpful principle of Stoicism, which is also found in Buddhism, is this, from Epictetus's *Enchiridion*:

"Freedom and happiness consist of understanding one principle: There are certain things we can control and certain things we cannot control. It is only after learning to distinguish between what we can and cannot control – and acting upon that knowledge – that inner harmony and outer effectiveness become possible".[172]

If some of the things that negatively affect me, in my current social environment, are within my control, then it makes sense to try to correct and control them: to change them. And if something proves to be beyond my control - (or *most likely* beyond my control – including my ability to move to a new environment!) - then it makes sense not to rail against that, but *to learn to* **accept** it (which will take time and effort, and courage and fortitude).

But that is *not* (ultimately) what is taught by the major Stoic philosophers, when they deploy their more extreme principles.

For example, in his *Meditations*, Marcus Aurelius defines 'harm' as being the ability of some outside agency to damage his 'individual ethical stance'. And he then declares an absolute principle that: **Nobody has the ability to damage my individual ethical stance.** Hence, *logically*, nobody has the ability to **harm** him. Hence, his final conclusion: **Nobody can disturb me!**

(See the **Introduction** to the **Meditations**, by D.A. Ross)[173].

The problem with that conclusion is that only a rare sage could live a life based on the idea – the *fantasy* – that *a hatchet through my skull does not constitute* <u>harm</u>*, since it leaves my individual ethical stance intact.*

Or, that somebody murdering my baby and raping my wife cannot disturb me, *because it leaves my individual ethical stance intact.*

These are *unreachable* goals, and *inhuman* beliefs, which could never be *universalized* as an approach to life. And therefore, counsellors and psychotherapists should not (morally) imply that these are goals which are achievable by average counselling clients; and that the client is somehow remiss for not acting like a lump of wood!

~~~

So, while we can learn some things about *moderating our desires* and *distinguishing* between what is a *realistic* goal (to be pursued) and an *unachievable* goal (to be abandoned) – we must not spread *the lie that our clients are* <u>not</u> *disturbed by their social experiences! They* <u>are</u>*!* (See above, for a description of the *six or more factors* which - jointly - cause human disturbance - one of which is the External Activating Event [A1], which is to say, *what happens* *to the individual* who then goes on to experience a consequent emotion!)

~~~

E3: Another point of departure – Evolutionary psychology

While Buddhism and Stoicism mainly apply *the **negative** theory of emotion* – which assumes that *all* emotions are problematical - evolutionary psychology promotes the idea that our emotions arose, and were selected by nature, because *they **served** to keep our ancestors alive*. This is a *positive* theory of emotion.

Evolutionary psychology is an attempt to build a science of psychology, based on inferences - (many from anthropological studies; and many which appear to be little more than applied logic, or philosophical thought experiments) - about the ways in which our ancestors adapted to their environments, and how and why some psychological adaptations were most likely selected by nature for their survival value. For examples:

Without your innate tendency towards anger, there would be nothing to stop selfish individuals taking advantage of you, even to the extent of threatening your survival (by stealing all the available food, for example).

Without anxiety, you might sit and watch with curiosity while a lion approached you and then ate you.

Without distress (or sadness) you might be unable to attract social support when you are weakened by illness, or when you are otherwise disadvantaged and in need of extra support.

Without feelings of lust and romantic love, you might fail to attract a mate; fail to reproduce yourself; and the quality of your life might seem so poor (relative to social norms) that you could easily abandon the attempt to stay alive.

So feelings - even apparently destructive or painful emotions - can be seen to serve useful survival functions, *except when they are taken **too far**, and then they cause more harm than good.*

And, paradoxically, as pointed out by Siegel (2015), emotions are both *regulated* and *regulatory*. They are regulated (or controlled) by both internal and external factors; and we also tend to internalize those external, social factors over time. (This external factor often takes the form of verbal or non-verbal feedback from significant others [mother, father, others] about their experience of our emotional expression [or expression of affects]).

Some of our emotive-cognitive experiences (including that feedback from significant others) help us to regulate other of our emotive-cognitive urges.

Another way to say this is as follows: We have our innate affects, or emotions, *socialized* by mother/father; and this shapes *our **subsequent capacity** to perfink* (or perceive-feel-think). Then, when some new event impinges upon our consciousness, we use our historical capacity to perfink to regulate our current perfinking response to this new experience. (Of course, this is *an exaggerated statement of 'agency'*. In fact, it is not *"us"* that does anything! It is not so much that "we use" our historical capacity to perfink; but rather that "we are used by" our historical capacity to perfink. It is rather more that *our historical **capacity** to perfink* – which is electro-chemical, body-brain-mind, culturally shaped memories - *automatically regulates our subsequent perfinking* about new and novel incoming stimuli).

While cognitive therapists elevate 'thinking' to the driving seat of human behaviour; and affect regulation theorists elevate 'feeling' to this role; we in emotive-cognitive (E-CENT) theory, attribute overall control of the body-brain-mind to **perfinking** – which is *integrated, interwoven, perceiving-feeling-thinking*; which is so hopelessly intertwined that *it is not possible to **separate** out the strands* from each other.

The **modelling** (or **demonstration**) of emotional self-regulation by our parents – as they engage in *their own **perfinking** performances* - is another of the major internalized sources of self-regulation that we have (which begins outside of us, but ends up encoded in our neurological, higher cognitive emotions, probably largely in the right orbitofrontal cortex [OFC]).

An example of the excessive use of negative emotions would be the driver who is so angry about being frustrated by other drivers that he (or she) gets out of their car and assaults somebody – killing or maiming them; resulting in great harm to both parties.

Or the person who is so anxious they cannot go out of their own home, and thus they miss out on all kinds of social pleasures (and the possibility of earning a living!)

Or somebody who is so distressed (sad/ depressed) that they cannot relate to others, and they lose their life partner as a result.

Some of these overly-emotional responses may come from our family of origin; and some may come from changes in our lives today, including in our relationships, our stress levels, our diets, or the balance/ harmony of our lives; or even from pharmaceutical drugs we take to 'cure' ourselves[174].

~~~

On balance, in E-CENT counselling, we see emotion as being more positive than negative, and more helpful than unhelpful – though it is obvious that our emotions can complicate our lives and cause us suffering when we do not manage them well.

~~~

But we still have not defined emotion, nor said anything about the origin of emotions in the historical processes of evolution of species.

E4: The origin of human emotions

Charles Darwin was the first major theorist to publish a serious study of the ways in which life on earth most likely evolved, and the principles that seem to control the evolutionary process – primarily *natural selection* of those *randomly arising features* of *organisms* which best fit an available ecological niche or habitat. Or, to state it in another way: Those organisms which were well adapted to survive in their local environment were the ones which survived to pass on their genes; and those who were poorly adapted did not survive.

Darwin noted, in his book on emotions in humans and other animals[175], that all mammals displayed similar emotional arousal patterns. This he saw as evidence for a common ancestor. But he considered that those emotions were a *residue* of more primitive times, while recent research suggests that **emotions are fundamental to all brain-mind functioning**, being **primary processes** which *modulate* cognitions (like attention, perception, thinking and memory processes); *generate* evaluations; *drive* goals; and *dictate* behaviours. (Panksepp, 1998).

Much later, Paul Ekman, an American anthropologist, set out to prove that Darwin was **wrong** about the *universality* of all basic primate and mammal emotions; and that, in fact, many cultures are wired up emotionally to be very *different* from each other – the major example being westerners versus the oriental mind. This is the famous (or *infamous!*) concept of 'cultural relativity'. However, despite the rigour of his studies, Ekman only succeeded in *proving Darwin to be **right**.* There is **no** *cultural relativity in respect of the **basic** human emotions* of anger, fear, distress, surprise, disgust and joy[176]. There are some cultural differences in *how* those emotions are **expressed** – for example the American and southern European tendency to be very open about feelings and emotions, on the one hand; and the Japanese tendency to be concealing of their feelings and emotions – but *the basic emotions – which are being revealed or concealed - are **common** to all cultures.*

~~~

Professor Jonathan Turner[177] has written an extensive study of the origins of human emotions. He draws attention to the *social* nature of humans and the relatively *solitary* practices of other kinds of apes; and argues that the development of our increased *sociality*[178] was brought about to facilitate living in the more exposed environment of the savannah, where *banding together* provided the best chance of survival. This need encouraged strong emotional ties, "allowing our ancestors to build higher levels of social solidarity". So *the social nature of human emotions* (or, rather, our higher cognitive emotions) can be explained in this way – as a constructive adaptation to a new foraging environment. But we still share our *basic emotions* with all mammals (as argued by Darwin and confirmed by Ekman, as mentioned above).

Jaak Panksepp is one of the foremost researchers in the field of affective neuroscience. In his book on the archaeology of mind, he "reveals for the first time the deep neural sources of our values and basic emotional feelings". These patterns in the human brain "are remarkably similar across all mammalian species"[179].

And we know from some brain studies that **some** emotional disorders result from damage to those emotional centres of the brain. However, **most** emotional disorders probably arise out of disruption of the *higher cognitive* and *social* emotions, (like guilt and pride), which will be introduced and discussed later.

~~~

...

E6: The evolutionary view

The perspectives of *evolutionary psychology* and *affective neuroscience* are better sources of explanation of human emotions. According to Panksepp and Biven (2012) our evolutionary adaptations (as mammals) laid down certain subcortical structures in the limbic areas of the brain. These neurological structures underpin seven emotional systems as follows:

1. **Seeking**: This emotional system is about how the brain generates a euphoric and expectant response. (I am wired up by nature to seek: human faces; comfort; food; and as I grow, to seek novelty, stimulation. (I 'want' what I am *programmed* by nature to 'want'!) So when I am 'wanting' many experiences, I am expressing an innate, biochemical urge laid down by natural selection. Of course, my list of wants can be, and is, expanded by my cultural conditioning and experience).

2. **Fear**: This system is about how the brain responds to the threat of physical danger and death. (I am wired up by nature [natural selection] to fear threats and dangers, because my ancestors who survived long enough to reproduce were kept alive by their fear of predators; and they passed that fear down the line, biochemically. This is my innate 'flight response'. I 'want' to survive, because I am programmed by nature of 'want' to survive! [Again, of course, I can learn to fear things that are not real threats or dangers]).

3. **Rage**: This system is about sources of irritation and fury in the brain. (I am wired up by natural selection to respond ragefully to serious frustrations, and to those threats and dangers in response to which I can overcome my natural fearfulness, presumably because this tendency in my ancestors helped to keep them alive long enough to reproduce. This is my innate 'fight response').

4. **Lust**: This system is about how sexual desire and attachments are elaborated in the brain. (I am wired up by natural selection to feel love and sexual desire. Without this lust and desire for sexual congress, and close physical comfort, my ancestors might not have bothered to reproduce, and I would not exist. Because they survived, they passed on their loving-lusting tendencies to me).

5. **Care**: This system is about sources of maternal nurturance. (Mothers do not 'decide' to care for their young. Among our ancestral tribes, any non-caring mothers - [who lacked a strong, innate caring urge], would have been

unlikely to keep their offspring alive long enough to reproduce, so non-caring attitudes tended to die out. Those mothers who kept their offspring alive long enough to reproduce were most likely those with neurologically wired tendencies to care sufficiently: to be 'good enough' mothers).

6. **Grief**: This system drives feelings of intense loss when I lose a significant 'attachment figure', whether they are sexual or non-sexual attachments. (I attach myself to significant others [especially mother {or my main carer}], by innate urging. This maximizes my chances of survival, so I can live to reproduce, and pass on to my offspring this same urge to attach to me and their other carers. But the downside of my strong attachment is that when my attachment figures die, or become unavailable to me, I experience an intense sense of loss [grief]). This is also the foundation of sadness and depression.

7. **Play**: This urge explains how the brain generates joyous, rough-and-tumble interactions. (I have innate urges to play, driven by a sense of joy in my own playfulness, and the responses of my playmates. This may have survived through evolutionary time because my playfulness makes me attractive to my carers, and so they want to protect me to keep me alive and near them. Less playful and joyful children might have been abandoned in tough times, and so their less-playful genes died out).

~~~

The general point arising out of Panksepp's research on the brains of animals, and other studies, is that all mammals have these seven basic emotional systems hardwired into the limbic system (or mammalian brain). These seven systems probably should not be seen as the end of the matter, since Panksepp himself included *panic* in his original list, and omitted *grief.*

The take-home message seems to be this: Every human being is carrying a set of basic emotional, motivational and automatic control systems (or the developmental capacity to create them) in the subcortical areas of their brains, at birth. Their neocortex, on the other hand, is available to be wired up by social encounters. Their social encounters, initially, are managed from their basic emotions, which, through social interactions become woven together with social experiences, into 'higher cognitive emotions'. This most likely takes place in the right orbitofrontal cortex, where the limbic system and the neocortex overlap. (Hill, 2015).

Contrary to Albert Ellis's view, *emotion,* on the one hand, and *conscious thought,* on the other, begin as two **separate**, brain-based systems, which interact and moderate each other, so that reason (when it emerges over developmental time in the child) **depends upon** basic emotions [in the limbic system], (plus socially influenced emotions [based in the orbitofrontal cortex]), which are required to evaluate (value) the significance of thoughts, options, actions, etc. (Siegel, 2015; Damasio, 1994).

Logic **cannot** tell us what to value, what to like, or what to love (Damasio, 1994)[180]. Those evaluations are made by our emotional systems (including our basic emotions and our higher cognitive emotions, including our moral emotions of guilt, shame and elevation [Haidt, 2006]).

E7: Understanding emotive-cognitive interactionism

Before we move on to look at the *socialization of emotion,* as discussed in interpersonal neurobiology (Siegel, 2015)[181], let us review the E-CENT model of mind as developed in one of our main papers in 2009[182].

In this paper I reviewed the main theory of REBT regarding the connection between thinking and emotions.

Albert Ellis began (in the mid-1950's) with the thesis that thinking, feeling and action were all *interconnected,* and in many respects *essentially the same thing.*[183]

In Figure 2 of Byrne (2009c), which is reproduced in Figure E.2 below, I presented the classic ABC model of REBT, with the embellishment that, at point B, in the middle of the model, I showed:

B1 = Emotive processing (quick, primary)

B2 = Cognitive processing (slow, secondary)

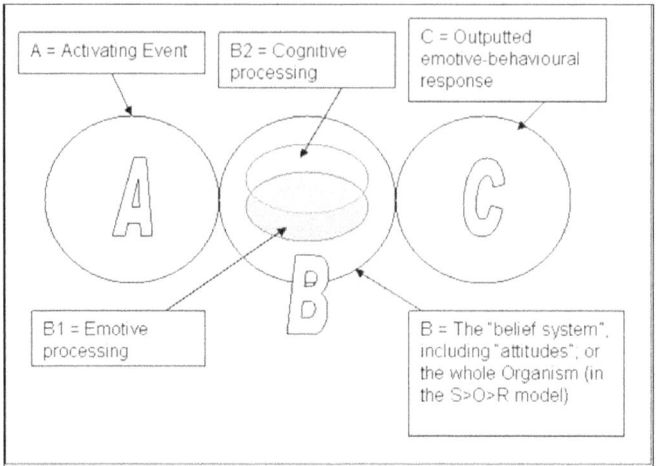

Figure 2: The overlapping of thinking and feeling in Ellis (1958)

Figure E2: The interaction of thinking and feeling in the complex ABC model

And B1 and B2 are shown to be partially overlapping, to reflect Albert Ellis's claim that thinking and feeling are interactional and partly-overlapping in nature.

However, now, in the light of Panksepp and Biven (2012) and other modern sources on neurobiology, I want to amend that to say this:

The individual human has innate emotional control systems in their limbic system, which are relatively standardized.

If we take the example of a seven year old boy, he also has, by this stage of his development, acquired some limited cognitive processing capabilities based (or managed from) his frontal lobes.

And what we used to call the overlapping aspects of B1 (emotion) and B2 (thinking) we now see as being the ways in which his limbic system and his frontal lobes *interact*.

And, from the time of his birth, those interactions will have been strongly influenced by his social relationships, especially with mother (and later father and others).

What follows is an illustration of how Panksepp (1998) lists the elements of, and lines of communication between, a stimulus and a human response.

See Figure E.3 below:

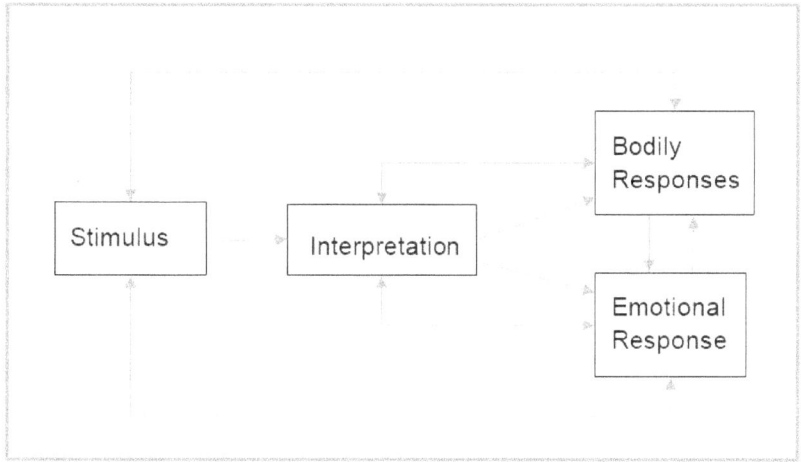

Figure E3: From a presentation by Jaak Panksepp (Slide 12)[184]

This one of several ways to conceptualize the relationship between an organism and its environmental stimuli. And it is probably the most complete, and convincing model I've seen.

At the very least, we would claim that the incoming stimulus is interpreted, on the basis of the organism's innate wiring, and its memorized experiences. That interpretation triggers both a bodily response and an emotional (feeling, or affect) response. (Indeed, it would be more accurate to say: The interpretation is *both* (a) triggered by past physical-emotional experiences, and (b) triggers new, similar physical-emotional responses in the present moment).

The bodily response and the emotional response communicate with each other and send signals back to the interpretation, which will tend to modify it.

The bodily response and emotional response may also change the stimulus, (for example: if the stimulus is a comprehending being that reads body language and facial expressions).

The E-CENT perspective (in Figure E4 below) accords with – or overlaps and lines up with - the model by Jaak Panksepp, in Figure E3 above.

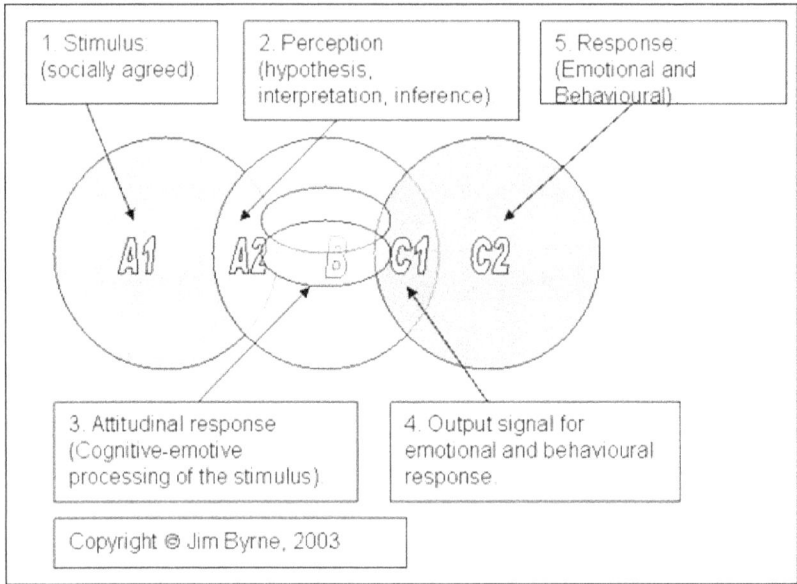

Figure E4: Further elaboration of the complex ABC model

That is to say, as we see it: A stimulus (A1) is interpreted (at A2) and that interpretation sets off a pattern-matched set of bodily and facial responses, as well as innate and socially shaped emotional responses.

Those responses feed back to the interpretation, to refine, modify or intensify it, and a feed-back signal goes to the bodily responses and the emotional responses to modulate them.

As the emotional state stabilizes, the higher cognitive functions (reflective thinking/ feeling/ appraising) begin to kick in, and may radically modify the original interpretation.

This model is predicated upon (or based upon) well known and reliably inferred interactions between the various elements of the neocortex and the limbic system. And this is a change from Figure E2 above.

The ABC model in Figure E4 was influenced by both Ellis (1958, 1962) and also Damasio (1994).

Ellis described thinking and feeling as overlapping, and Damasio (1994) seemed to suggest that there was an area of the frontal lobes where reasoning and emotion interacted and moderated each other.

Now, it seems from Panksepp's anatomical studies, that rather than a 'place' where that happens, there are, instead, *a number of interactional connections between the emotional and reasoning centres of the brain*, which are themselves *discrete* and *separate* entities.

See Figure E5:

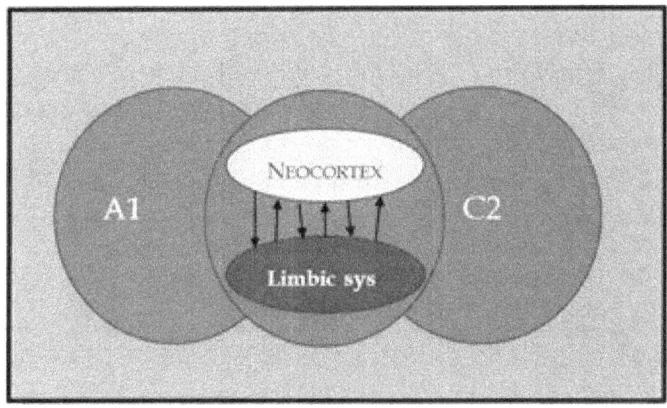

Figure E5: A new (hypothetical) model of the complex ABCs

This is one way to rethink the structures of cognitive-emotive functioning.

But there may still be a place where this happens, as suggested by Siegel (2015), which is the orbitofrontal cortex (or OFC).

In this new view, a stimulus in the external environment (A1) triggers an interpretation/inference/pattern-match, in the limbic system (initially), which – if the stimulus is sufficiently strong (for example, frightening) causes a signal to be sent (via the limbic system) to C1 (the 'output-manager' or 'action-controller') to take immediate defensive or self-protective action, as argued by LeDoux (1998)[185]. On the other hand, if the stimulus is sufficiently non-urgent, then a slower route towards forming a response is taken, via the neocortex and the individual's history of similar situations (again as clarified by LeDoux, 1998).

From the point of view of a counsellor sitting with a client in their counselling room, the take away message is this:

For most practical purposes, the client is more like a stimulus-response organism than not. They have *emotive-cognitive processing* going on at point B in the ABC model, but that is either handled by their automatic limbic instincts, or by their habitual patterns of response, laid down by their social history, which is most likely managed from the orbitofrontal cortex.

And we may be able to sustain the original idea of the overlapping areas of thinking and emotion, if we accept the description of the orbitofrontal cortex in the writings of Jaak Panksepp (see Panksepp and Biven, 2012). Panksepp describes the orbitofrontal cortex as a prefrontal cortex region in the frontal lobes of the brain which is involved in the cognitive processing of decision making. *But it is also considered to be a **part of the limbic system**.* If it belongs to both the limbic system and the frontal lobes, then is seems like the kind of entity described in the 'overlapping' of brain functions and brain areas.

~~~

Daniel Siegel (2015) suggests a tripartite model of the human 'individual', in which the brain of a child, interacting with its mother, gives rise to 'mind'. This is very similar to the basic E-CENT model which will be reviewed below, but which is essentially about the ways in which the mind of the baby and mother interpenetrate and give rise to the 'ego' or personality of the child.

Daniel Hill's (2015) description suggests a broader, four-part model of human functioning which looks like Figure E.6 below. This new model by Hill suggests that, far from language, or thoughts, or beliefs being the intervening factor between a person's experience of challenges in their environment and their emotional/ behavioural response, the emotional limbic system seems like a better candidate for this role, given its centrality to the organism-environment whole.

This is it:

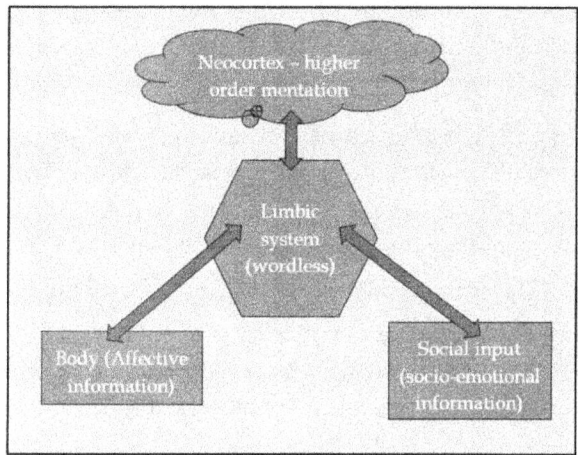

Figure E6: Daniel Hill's (2015) four-part model

The wordless limbic system was our original (emotional) control centre, and it continues to be in ultimate control, and it continues to be wordless.

But the overlapping area with the neocortex, the orbitofrontal cortex (OFC), should be seen to store *social learning*, much of which was derived from *language-based instruction*. And if my personality (or 'ego') has a physical (electro-chemical and hormonal base) then it most likely is my orbitofrontal cortex (OFC). (See Damasio on Elliott, in Damasio, 1998).

E8: Language and mentation

With regard to Daniel Hill's (2015) emphasis upon the *wordlessness* of the limbic system, I should emphasize that the orbitofrontal cortex, which is most likely the seat of the personality and character – the ego – must be assumed to be wired up by *an integration of socialized experience* (including language, actions and paralinguistics) with the innate emotional control systems. (Mahrabian, 1981)[186].

This would mean that, although therapists' nonverbal, emotional communications are very important, so also are their statements, pronouncements and actions in the world.

The client *interprets* what the counsellor or therapist does and says. And those interpretations are largely automatic and non-conscious. Some small elements may enter consciousness.

If the client spots a contradiction between the counsellor's words and the counsellor's actions, s/he will most likely trust the actions and discount the words.

The client interprets what the counsellor says and does, on the basis of their past experiences. They may discount words which they found, earlier in life, to be hollow, or insincere. If they are not accustomed to kind words, or praising words, they may discount them. They may discount anything that they have previously decided to be untrue; or untrue about themselves.

Just as the client *perfinks* – or perceives, feels and thinks – all in one grasp of the mind; so the counsellor must be seen to *communicate* – or to speak, act and metalinguistically emote – all in one act of the self.

And the counsellor does not *know (precisely)* **what** s/he is communicating to the client, because:

(a) S/he is a habit-based, socialized, organic being (which is what *all humans* are!). S/he is a largely non-conscious, automatic, stimulus-response organism, just like the client – except a good therapist has been trained to respond as a helpful person. And:

(b) The client interprets the counsellor's words and actions in the light of the client's own experiences, and not in the light of a glossary of the counsellor's meanings!

However, a good, holistic counsellor often knows the kind of being she is, and therefore gets adequate sleep and hydration and exercise and nutrition (and perhaps meditation) before coming to a counselling session.

Furthermore, a good counsellor should have a better 'map of the good life' to share with the client, who most often has a *dysfunctional map* of life.

And both of those life maps include non-verbal experiences, emotional-cognitive responses, and linguistically-derived elements.

Finally, that brings us neatly to the *social model* of the individual, which I also developed in 2009.

E9: The social individual

After reviewing the complex ABC model, I went on to lay down the basic E-CENT model of the mother-baby dyad, in Figure 5 of Byrne (2009b)[187], as shown in Figure E.7 below.

This model helped us to explore the ways in which the mother of a new-born baby has to colonize the baby; take it over; and run its life, for the sake of its survival. The first couple of years of each of our lives is spent in close proximity to mother (or a substitute carer), who is more or less sensitive to our needs; more or less responsive, attuned, and timely in responding; more or less gentle and caring; and so on.

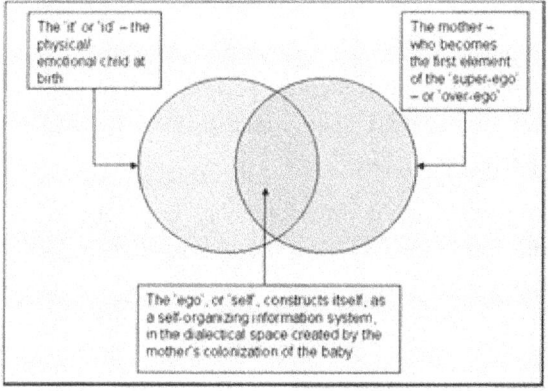

Figure E7: The most basic model of E-CENT counselling theory

The personality of the mother dictates the kind of care we get; and the kind of care that we got is internalized as the foundations of our first *Internal Working Model* of relationship. If she can provide us with a 'secure base', then we will grow up with a secure sense of attachment to subsequent love objects, including the individual(s) we marry[188].

Next I will present an important model from Transactional Analysis (TA).

It may be that the OK-Corral from Transactional Analysis (TA) captures the core decision of significance which is at the centre of the *Internal Working Model.*

This is how the OK-corral model looks:

		Your Decision About Others	
		OK	Not-OK
Your Decision About Yourself	OK	1. I'm OK - You're OK	2. I'm OK - You're Not-OK
	Not-OK	3. I'm Not-OK - You're OK	4. I'm Not-OK - You're Not-OK

Figure E8: The OK Corral from TA

Thus my basic decision about my relationship with mother might be this: "I'm okay, and so is she!" But it could equally be that "I'm not okay, but she is!" And so on. That early decision, about who I am and how I feel valued or devalued, marks me for life!

This model can be translated (theoretically; propositionally) into a *Working Model equivalent*, in the form of **adult attachment styles**, like this:

		Thoughts-feelings about self	
		Positive	Negative
Thoughts-feelings about partner	Positive	**Secure:** (comfortable with intimacy and autonomy)	**Preoccupied:** (Anxious-ambivalent about relationship: Clingy)
	Negative	**Dismissing:** (Avoidant attachment, cool and remote)	**Disorganized:** (Confused, dissociating, blanking out: Approach-avoidance)

Figure E9: Adult attachment styles and appraisals of self and others

This is not a perfect fit with attachment theory, but it has some useful features, and some caveats. For example, the **preoccupied** mind-set of the anxious-ambivalent individual is based on a negative view of the self (or at least a view of the self as *not self-sufficient*, and of *desperately* needing the other person to stick around). And this causes their tendency to cling. On the other hand, they may not see their partner as 'positive' as such (and they may even cling angrily!) but they view their partner as a *'positive **asset'*** to which they must hold on!

We can also infer, in the average case, that if the mother's (and father's [or main carer's]) way of relating to the baby results in a positive self-appraisal (which is emotive-cognitive), and in a positive appraisal of the care provided by the main carer, then the baby (and later adult) will form a **secure** attachment style, in which they are comfortable with intimacy and autonomy.

On the other hand, in the absence of good-enough parenting, the individual is likely to develop an avoidant, or anxious-ambivalent, or disorganized attachment style.

Of course, there is more to attachment styles than is suggested here.

In particular, each individual builds up a non-linguistic, non-conscious picture of *"How 'they' related to me;* **who** *that 'makes me'; and how I had to relate to 'them'; and how I must relate to any new (significant) person in front of (adult) me today."*

We do not have to think about any of this. It's all automatic and non-conscious; a set of pre-patterned ways of relating, based on foundational experiences.

~~~

It takes five or six months for us to distinguish ourselves from our mothers, and we rely upon her, not just for food and comfort and taking care of our colic, and changing our soiled clothing, and so on; but also, and perhaps much more importantly, for her ability *to sooth our **uncontrollable** emotions.*

Young babies cannot soothe themselves, and need external assistance with this challenge. As we grow up, we take back some of those controls, but we never completely outgrow the need for external assistance with 'affect regulation'. (Lewis, Amini, and Lannon, (2001))[189]. We need our mothers to love us if our socialized brains are to grow and provide us with an adequate measure of social and emotional intelligence (Gerhardt, 2010)[190].

As mother interacts with her baby, the baby internalizes representations of the experience of those encounters – at least those which seem emotionally significant. (Siegel, 2015)[191]. And out of those encounters, the baby constructs its *ego*, or *personality* (as illustrated in Figure E.7 above).

As I wrote at that time:

"Thus the mother wires up the brain of her baby, initially by handling and managing its body; and later by introducing the baby to her language, her linguistic culture, her rules, and her language-based world." (Byrne, 2009b).

But today I would also want to add this: It is not all about language and culture. It is also about the mother's behaviours, and the child's interpretation of those behaviours; which show up as both *narrativized* and *non-narrativized experiences*!

Of course, the baby brings something to the party – his or her innate wiring in the brain stem and the limbic system; and its enteric brain (in its guts). All of which is instinctive and emotional. There are no 'innate beliefs', since 'beliefs' are linguistic constructions.

So, it is more useful to see the ABC/SOR/EFR models differently. The major mediating variable between

(1) new Activating Stimuli – coming into the senses of the child – and

(2) outgoing emotional and behavioural responses,

can now be seen to be

(3) **Experiences**, and **not** Beliefs!

That is to say, we are wired up for today by our **Previous Experiences**, from the past; *some of which have been* **narrativized** (or can be articulated in language today); and *some of which were* **never narrativized**, and cannot be accessed today - because they are totally non-conscious, and beyond retrieval. But they nevertheless play a role in *guiding* *our reactions* to new events today!

~~~

I have argued above that there are seven innate emotional control systems, and there is an evaluation capacity – 'good' – 'bad' – which guides the baby's reactions to incoming stimuli. A felt experience seems either negative or positive to the new-born baby and young infant; and this triggers one of the emotional control systems: (e.g. anger or fear, or joy, etc.)

The baby, as it develops, shows signs of having pro- and anti-social tendencies, but these are shaped overwhelmingly by the mother's level of skill. A skilful mother can soothe a truculent baby; while an unskilful mother can aggravate and irritate a calm baby and render it truculent.

As the baby grows and encounters mother and father and perhaps a sibling or two, and perhaps *granny*, and *babysitters*, and then perhaps *nursery teachers*, and so on, s/he increasingly internalizes their ways of being: their Parental tendencies; their Adult tendencies; their Child-like tendencies.

And the child can also link those states to its own child-like tendencies, and, from age two years onwards, increasingly to act like a Little Professor, asking questions and exploring its environment.

But s/he (the child) mainly learns from instruction and modelling, and trial and error, and eventually can organize all those Parent, Adult and Child experiences – with good and bad aspects – into coherent wholes, below the level of conscious awareness, until his or her personality (C) emerges (through the interaction of A and B) like this:

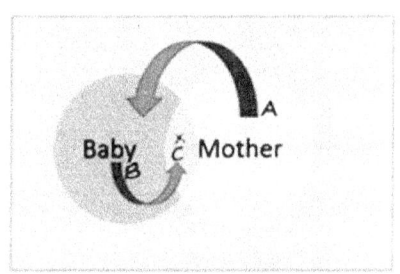

The child internalizes representations of its encounters with mother, and in the overlapping space of encounter, a cluster of ego state possibilities arise, which are later triggered by external stimuli. (See Figure E.10 below). And in the overlapping space of their emotional encounters, the child constructs its own sense of self.

The child knows how to act like the child it is today, and the child it was in an earlier period (regressing to that state when stress levels are high).

The child knows how mother and father act and speak.

So children know not just *how to be scientific* and *inquiring*, and *how to be playful*, but also *how to order mother* to do things, and *how to comfort mother* when she is apparently unwell.

(In other words, children have a number of *different* embryonic ego-states, or ways of being, which they copied from their social environment; and which we commonly call **Parent Adult** and **Child** ego states).

See Figure E10, below:

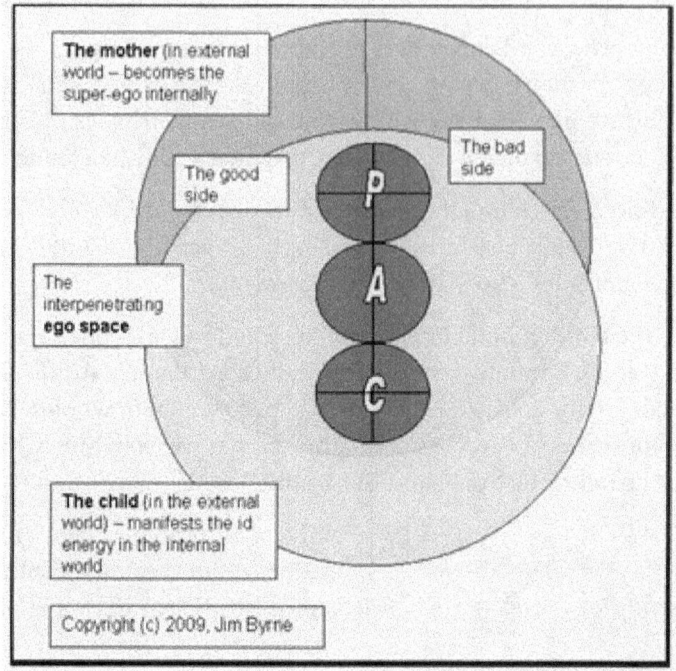

Figure E10: The structure of the child's ego

Each of those 'ego state' possibilities – Child, Parent, Adult - has a **good** side and a **bad** side. The good side is constructive and pro-social; and the bad side is destructive and anti-social. (These two states are also known as *Eros* and *Thanatos* [in Freud's language] – or the *Good Wolf* and the *Bad Wolf* [in the language of the native American Cherokee people]).

Figure E.10 above shows a summary of those developments.

The emergent ego of every child contains the embryonic components of Good and Bad Nurturing Parent; Good and Bad Controlling Parent; Good and Bad Adult; Good and Bad Adapted/Rebellious Child; and Good and Bad Free (or Natural) Child.

~~~

In Byrne (2009b), I explored the nature of a physical/social human by exploring my own nature. This was my conclusion:

Perhaps I am just this physical organism (body/brain/mind)

Including its feeling/affective foundation (in the limbic system)

And its language based – or language-aided - cognitive/emotive superstructure (in the neocortex, and the orbitofrontal cortex)

With all of its cumulative, interpretative experiences

Including internalized representations of good and bad aspects of significant others

And all of my good and bad adaptations towards them

And my good and bad reactions and rebellions against them

Which gave rise to my Internal Working Models, of how they (my significant others) related to me (positively or negatively), and how I related to them (positively or negatively)

All of which is stored in long term memory

*In the form of electro-chemical equivalents of stories, scripts, frames, schemas and other narrativized **and non-narrativized** elements*

Below the level of conscious awareness

*And **permanently** beyond direct conscious inspection.*

Perhaps that is what I most fundamentally am. And thus, although I am *distinct* from others, I carry many others inside my head, and I am indeed made up of many 'social/ relational/ interactional bits and pieces'. So I am both individual and social. But I am very far from being a 'separate entity'.

Because my sense of 'self' develops in lockstep with my sense of 'society', and with my biological development, none of these three 'levels' of 'me/I/us' can exist (for any significant period of time) without the other.

~~~

From the point of view of an E-CENT counsellor, working with a client, it is important to note that the individual is hard-wired by nature to be *an emotional being*. This emotional being (as a baby) is thrown into a family with its own cultural shape, which impacts the baby so powerfully that it leaves its mark on the baby like a die stamps a pattern on a copper or silver coin. The coin is malleable, and can be melted down and re-stamped, but not easily. (It takes a lot of heat to melt it!) And the child, once grown up, retains some neurological and psychological malleability, but also lots of rigidity or habit-based inflexibilities.

Counselling and therapy can begin to work on restructuring the emotional/ neurological shape of the socialized individual (by 'melting it'), but the outcome depends upon how good the client is at taking on the necessary hard work (of melting into the possibilities offered – many of which will involve feeling previously unfelt pains!).

The counsellor can be available as a secure base for the client - and a safe harbour to come back to again and again - and thus hope to re-parent the client (which also means: *to re-educate the emotions and thinking* of the client). But none of this is easy, and it's certainly not automatic.

When a client sits before me, I do not see a discrete, separate, stand-alone individual. I see the outworking of a complex family history. I sense the many Internal Working Models from which this social-individual relates to the world. I am aware that this is *an emotional being*, with some capacity to *think* (or *perfink*!) and learn; but also most likely s/he is a "community of sub-personalities"[192] with some strongly *frozen **schemas**!* Those 'frozen schemas' are fixed *frames*, or ways of perceiving-feeling-thinking about the world as interpreted. And, because those frames are non-conscious, the client cannot offer them up for examination in counselling. They have to be 'stumbled upon' by serendipity!

~~~

Let us now look at how we can tackle some typical emotional disturbances - like anger, anxiety and depression - in counselling or self-help contexts.

E10: Managing human emotions

Like Panksepp (1998)[193] and Schore (2015)[194], Daniel Siegel in his (2015) book on the developing mind, emphasizes that what we call 'appraisal' is an *emotive* rather than a **thinking** process. The emotional centres of the brain can appraise an incoming stimulus as either 'good' or 'bad' from the beginning of life, long before we have any form of language labels. (This has been tested empirically, with either a sweet or a sour drink for the baby's first drink after birth, combined with observation of their facial responses!)[195] And from this innate appraisal process, and using our emotional control systems (described by Panksepp, 1998), we elaborate some basic emotional reactions, of anger, sadness, fear, surprise and/or joy[196].

In E-CENT theory we see that slightly differently.

In the beginning, the baby uses its innate, basic emotions to evaluate the goodness or badness of a situation.

But over time, and especially in the first two or three years of life, the new child is taught by its carers to modulate its affects – through rewards, penalties, modelling, soothing, and so on, and it may be that that integration of socialized-emotions, or higher cognitive-emotions, are stored in the Orbitofrontal Cortex (OFC).

Thereafter, appraisal becomes *a learned emotive-cognitive process*. And it should be thought of as a function of *perfinking*, rather than either *thinking* (which is the CBT preference) or *emoting* (which is the Affect Regulation Theory preference).

Thus it is clear that E-CENT does not follow either of the extremes – the *cognitivists* or the *emotivists* – but rather that we have *'perfinked'* our own way to a *novel, balanced* solution, which takes account of the innate (emotive) affects, and the later (linguistic-cultural) shaping, both of which are woven together into the *perfinking body-brain-mind*.

~~~

Siegel's (2015) argument is that the baby's 'primary feelings' - (which can be expressed by us as 'this is good'; 'this is bad'; or 'this feels good'; 'this feels bad') – are elaborated over time into (categorical) emotions (of anger, sadness, joy, fear, etc.).

Furthermore, babies need external regulation (soothing), and it's the quality, quantity and timeliness of that soothing that shapes the baby's dominant mood and habitual emotional profile. (Siegel, 2015, page 183).

As we grow and develop, interact with our care-givers, learn to read their nonverbal emotional states, and increasingly acquire language, we also evolve/ acquire higher cognitive emotions (like guilt, shame, pride, love, embarrassment, elevation, envy, and jealousy, etc.): and the flow of basic emotions, and socially-shaped emotions, is what *creates meaning in our lives*, and allows us to appraise our situations in life. According to Siegel (2015): Emotions do not follow from thinking. Thinking follows from socialized-emotion.   Attention and perception are also modulated by emotion. Emotions are basic to who we are and who we become.   And the central features of emotion are *(non-conscious) appraisal* and *(non-conscious) arousal*. (Siegel, 2015. Pages 184-185).

Our ability to manage our emotions, to "regulate our affects", is a function of our history of attachment with our primary carers and subsequent significant others. (Bowlby, 1988/2005; Schore, 2015; Siegel, 2015; Wallin, 2007[197]).

In E-CENT theory, we see that slightly differently. Firstly, innate feelings precede, and are the foundation for, subsequent socialized perfinking (perceiving-feeling-thinking). What we call 'thinking' never was a separate function of the brain-mind. *It is one of our delusions* (Gray, 2003) that we are thinking being; that we think; that we have thoughts; that we can reason, separately and apart from feelings and automatic perceptions!

To an E-CENT counsellor, a client has two major aspects:

First, s/he is:

(1) A *physical/cultural organism*, with all of his/her cumulative, interpretive (*perfinked*) experiences, stored in long-term memory, below the level of conscious awareness, and permanently beyond conscious inspection: (Byrne 2009b). But the client is *also:*

(2) A *subjective*, felt-being, and feeling-being, a *virtual self* which feels like a *concrete* reality in the world. (Erwin, 1997)[198].

I do not *think* it ethical – or *perfink it* to be ethical - that we relate to the client exclusively on the basis of aspect (1) above. We must always recognize aspect (2) as *the dominant **reality** for the client*; while aspect (1) is the dominant reality for science.

But although E-CENT counsellors use science to find our way through the swamp of social and individual psychology, *we are **not** primarily scientists*.

*We are primarily **healers** and **feeling – perfinking** - beings*. We not only show our clients cognitive empathy (like all other systems of counselling and therapy) but also emotive empathy. We feel for the client; and with the client: (as do 'affect regulation' therapists – Hill, 2015).

And our obvious pain upon learning of the client's suffering is part of what heals them! (Because they 'feel felt'!)

We care deeply about our clients, because there is "only one being", and we all participate in that being. The universe is one big living being!

And then – if it is possible to anticipate what we normally do' - we try to get the client to tell us what is going on (confession) and we investigate that situation (explication), and then we set about educating the client, like a good parent – a good *re-parenting* 'secure base'.

In between the *explication* and the *education*, is the process of 'agreeing a story' of 'what is going on', or 'what is going wrong', which makes sense to us and to the client, *so we can **agree** a **potential** way forward.*

~~~

E11: Managing anger, anxiety and depression

So let us look, briefly, at those three common emotional problems mentioned above.

E11(a). Anger:

The E-CENT theory of anger says that anger is one of our basic emotions. It's innate. It was selected by nature for its survival value. We would not survive for long without an innate sense of *angering* in response to abuse or neglect. We also would not survive for long if we did not quickly learn how to *moderate* our anger as young children. My anger is a two-edged sword. It can help to protect me, and it can attract hostile reactions from others.

My **basic** emotion of anger is elaborated into a *higher cognitive emotion* through modelling by my mother and father and significant others in the first few years of my life. My ability to become *emotionally intelligent* in relation to my innate anger urges depends on the emotional intelligence of my parents. My first angry outbursts are with them. How successfully I and they handle those angry episodes will shape how I manage my anger in the school playground. And my socialized anger management strategies continue to evolve through my successful and my unsuccessful experiences of engaging in conflict with others: siblings, school peers, and so on.

I may become an *exploder*, who erupts in the faces of others. I may become an *imploder*, who keeps his anger inside. Or I may hide my anger from myself (repress it) and then project it into my environment where it may frighten me.

So anger is a socialized emotion, and if you grew up with angry people, you are likely to be prone to angering yourself when provoked; or you might feel fearful of your own anger, or the anger of others.

~~~

Healthy anger is present-time defence of your legitimate rights in the face of inappropriate behaviour by another person. Healthy or *reasonable* anger is the fuel that drives our **assertive** behaviours. It pushes us to engage in *constructive conflict*, when that is *necessary*!

To ask for what you want, which is legitimately yours to request, requires a certain level of 'fire in your belly'. If you lack that fire (that *reasonable* level of anger), then you will tend to 'wimp-out'; to act passively and let other people control you, or intimidate you, or deny you your reasonable share of the social stage. One of the problems that we encounter in therapy is this: Some parents, anxious to socialize their children to be 'nice' and 'civilized', go too far in 'switching off their fierceness' – instead of teaching them to manage their fierceness appropriately. And one of the things we do for passive clients is to help them to switch on their 'fierceness switch' – but to only use their fierceness assertively, up to the boundary of their personal space – and never to invade the personal space of another – or to use their fierceness aggressively!

Unhealthy or *unreasonable* anger is an over-reaction to a frustrating or insulting stimulus from another person or external force. Unhealthy or unreasonable anger leads to **aggressive** actions and destructive conflict. It is an excessive use of fierceness, and an under-use of communication and negotiation strategies.

We teach the following eight insights to our anger management clients:

1. You were born with *an **innate capacity** to develop angry*, anxious and depressed responses to your social environment - in response to frustrations, threats and losses.

2. You then encountered your mother, who already had a 'style of relating', based on her attachment experience of her own mother and father. She would inevitably have shaped your emotional expression by:

(a) Modelling an approach to relationship and emotions; and:

(b) Rewarding and penalizing you for your daily emotion expressions, including your angry outbursts in the first couple of years of your life.

3. Your father's approach to relationship, including emotion expression, especially his way of expressing (or suppressing) anger, would have been the next major influence on the development of your emotion expression, including your way of being angry - implosive or explosive; appropriate or inappropriate.

4. If both of your parents had a secure attachment to their own parents, they would have had a warm but assertive approach to relating to you. From them you would have learned to be secure in your relationship with them, and, by extension, in virtually all subsequent people-encounters. You would have learned to express healthy or appropriate anger in an *assertive* way - to ask for what you want, and to say no to what you do not want. And to strive to be treated with respect as an equal human being. You would not have any significant problems with anger.

5. However, if one or both of your parents had an insecure attachment to their own parents, they would have had an insecure attachment to you, and been either explosively or implosively angry with you when you frustrated them or broke their *personal* rules, or their *culturally shaped moral rules*. From them, you would have learned to engage in unhealthy or inappropriate anger expression of an explosive or implosive type, or a mixture of the two, varying from situation to situation. (Or you might have learned to be *passive* in those situations in which you felt frightened or fearful of reprisals, but *aggressive* in those situations where you felt no constraint of fearfulness!)

6. If you want to change your relationship style today, you need to experience secure relationship with another person - possibly a romantic partner; a very good friend; or a good therapist who understands how to build a secure relationship with you. You need to learn the difference between *appropriate* and *inappropriate* anger. And also that **explosive** anger - (like shouting and using aggressive body language) - costs you, in terms of damage to relationships and careers, for examples; and that *implosive anger* – (like sulking and stewing in your own angry juices, or withdrawing aggressively) - damages your ongoing happiness, your relationships at home and at work, and ultimately your physical and mental health.

7. You can improve your relationship and attachment style by studying and applying new ideas from emotional literacy and self-assertion. And I (and/or other counsellors) can teach those ideas and skills to you.

8. But you are also a body-mind, and so your approach to managing your diet, physical exercise, sleep pattern, self-talk (or inner dialogue), and relaxation/ meditation, are also important. And it is easier to develop a secure attachment style if your romantic partner is already secure.

~~~

When an E-CENT counsellor works with an angry client, they may work on deep, emotional and attachment issues from early childhood; or on present-time assertiveness skills; or advice on important dietary changes; or recommendations regarding regular physical exercise, or improvements to sleep patterns; or teaching the client how to reframe their anger-inducing experiences; or changing some elements of their philosophy of life (as they show up in their inner dialogues about anger-inducing situations) – and even to change some aspect of their social or physical environment with which they have been putting up or tolerating unnecessarily!

~~~

E12: Managing anger with diet and nutrition

In Taylor-Byrne and Byrne (2017), we explored - among other things - the key ways in which *diet can influence anger*. Some of the key findings were as follows:

Firstly, (unlike in the case of depression) there is at least one study which supports the idea that there is a link between low serotonin levels and the expression of anger, annoyance and irritation (specifically, low serotonin was linked to a reduced ability to self-manage rising levels of anger). We also presented evidence which showed that 5HTP, a natural nutritional supplement (from a West African medicinal plant called *Griffonia simpicifolia*), can be effective in restoring serotonin, an important neurotransmitter within the brain, thus reducing the expression of angry and hostile behaviour, as evidenced by Julie Ross's (2002) case study example.

The levels of copper and manganese in the client's body can have an effect on levels of anger; so vitamin and mineral supplementation seems to be important to address.

The link between violent behaviour - by young offenders (in prison) - and the condition known as 'reactive hypoglycaemia' (where blood sugar levels fall too low after eating high carbohydrate meals) - has been established by scientific research. There is thus an obvious connection between fluctuating blood sugar levels and anger management problems, and this can guide us in recommending particular (low sugar, slow-burning) foods to our angry clients.

A number of studies have established a definite link between a reduction in the consumption of sugar and refined foods, (on the one hand), and anger and anti-social behaviour, (on the other). In a similar vein, reductions in diets containing trans-fats, mainly involving hydrogenated fats in processed foods, led to a reduction in impatience, irritability and aggression in research participants.

Conversely, the link between pro-social behaviour and a healthy diet has also been evidenced by research. Dietary changes which increase the nutritional content of people's diets (especially introducing omega-3 fatty acids, as found for example in oily fish; plus vitamin and mineral supplements) result in improvements in pro-social behaviour, and better emotion and mood control. Anger levels declined in prisoners whose diet had been supplemented with fish oils, vitamins and minerals: and it has been shown that omega-3 fats have a rapid and significant impact on aggression in children and adults.

For further information, please see sections 4.3 to 4.7 above; and also Taylor-Byrne and Byrne (2017), for specific dietary guidance and advice.

~~~

E13: How anger can be reduced by exercise:

According to the British National Health Service website, anger is effectively reduced in intensity by exercising, including walking, swimming and yoga. Research studies have supported this view, and here are some examples which have provided valuable evidence on the role of exercise in anger reduction:

Research conducted by Joseph Tkacz, *et al.*, (2008), found that aerobic exercise regimes reduced anger expression among obese children. It was the first study which had been conducted to assess the value of having structured aerobic exercise sessions for overweight children, and the findings pointed to the value of exercise sessions after school.

Also, there was a study which investigated levels of anger amongst undergraduates at the University of Georgia. It looked at whether physical education (exercise) could moderate anger: (Reynolds, 2010); and it was reported in the *New York Times* magazine.

The 16 students selected were regularly oversensitive to provocations, and their anger was easily triggered.

They were subjected to different research conditions (*provocations*), designed to arouse their anger.

Firstly, those provocations were experienced without the benefits of exercise;

Secondly, they were experienced after the benefits of exercise.

The research results revealed that, the provocations had a stronger angering effect – producing a higher level of anger - *before* the exercise than they did after the participants had engaged in physical exercise.

After they had exercised, they were able to show composure and self-assurance in the face of emotional provocation. The physical exercise program did reduce their levels of anger, prompting the lead researcher, Nathaniel Thoms, a stress physiologist, to say:

"Exercise, even a single bout of it, can have a robust prophylactic (therapeutic) effect against the build-up of anger…it's like taking an aspirin to combat heart disease. You reduce your risk".

This result is echoed by the advice of the Mayo Clinic Staff, who have written that the higher the levels of stress a person is experiencing, the more likely they are to have high levels of anger, and that these effects can be diminished by vigorous and pleasurable exercise.

For further information, please see Appendix A, Section A2, above; plus Taylor-Byrne and Byrne (2017), for more specific information on research into different forms of exercise.

References

APA (2006) 'Forgiveness—Definitions and Effects'. Adapted from Philpot, C. (2006). Intergroup apologies and forgiveness. Unpublished PhD thesis, University of Queensland, Brisbane, Australia. Online: https://www.scribd .com/document/ 328941790/forgiveness-pdf. Accessed: 30th November 2018.

Armsden, G.C. and Greenberg, M.T. (1987) The inventory of parent and peer attachment: individual differences and their relationship to psychological well-being in adolescence. *Journal of Youth and Adolescence 16:* 427-454.

Aurelius, M. (1992). *Meditations*. Trans. by A.S.L. Farquharson. London: Everyman's Library.

Bandura, A., Ross, D., and Ross, S.A. (1961) Transmission of aggression through imitation of aggressive models. *Journal of Abnormal and Social Psychology, 63,* Pages 572-582.

Banyard, P. and Grayson, A. (2000) *Introducing Psychological Research: Seventy studies that shape psychology*. Second edition. Basingstoke, Hampshire: Palgrave.

Baran, J. (ed) (2003) *365 Nirvana: Here and now*. London: HarperCollins/Element.

Baskin and Enright (2004). 'Intervention studies on forgiveness: A meta-analysis.' *Journal of Counseling and Development 82*, 79-90.

Beck, C.J. (1997) *Everyday Zen: love and work*. London: Thorsons.

Beck, A.T. (1976/1989). *Cognitive Therapy and the Emotional Disorders.* London: Penguin Books.

Beck, A.T. (1999) *Prisoners of Hate: The Cognitive Basis of Anger, Hostility, and Violence*. New York: HarperCollins.

Ben-Shahar, T. (2007) *Happier: Learn the secrets to daily joy and lasting fulfilment.* New York: McGraw-Hill.

Bernstein, B. (1960) Language and social class. *British Journal of Sociology, 11,* 271-276.

Bernstein, B. (1961) Social class and linguistic development: A theory of social learning. In: A.H. Halsey, J. Floud and L.A. Anderson (eds) *Education, Economy and Society.* Glencoe: Free Press.

Blackburn, S. (1996) *Dictionary of Philosophy*. Oxford: Oxford University Press.

Bolton, R. (1979/1986). *People Skills: How to assert yourself, listen to others, and resolve conflicts.* Englewood Cliffs, NJ: Prentice-Hall Inc.

Bowlby, J. (1988/2005) *A Secure Base: clinical applications of attachment theory.* London: Routledge Classics.

Bretherton, I. (1992) The Origins of Attachment Theory: John Bowlby and Mary Ainsworth. *Developmental Psychology 28:* 759.

Briffa, J. (2005) 'High Anxiety', *Observer Magazine,* 19th June 2005, page 61.

Buddhism Online (2011) A view on Buddhism: Anger and Aversion. Available online: http:// viewon buddhism.org/anger.html. Accessed: 14th March 2011.

Burns, D. (1990) *The Feeling Good Handbook.* New York: Penguin/Plume.

Byrne, J. (2009a) A journey through models of mind. The story of my personal origins. E-CENT Paper No.4. Hebden Bridge: The Institute for E-CENT.

Byrne, J. (2009b) The 'Individual' and his/her Social Relationships - The E-CENT Perspective. E-CENT Paper No. 9. Hebden Bridge: The Institute for E-CENT. Available online: https://ecent-institute.org/e-cent-articles-and-papers/.

Byrne, J. (2009c) Rethinking the psychological models underpinning Rational Emotive Behaviour Therapy (REBT). E-CENT Paper No.1(a). Hebden Bridge: The Institute for E-CENT. Available online: https://ecent-institute.org/e-cent-articles-and-papers/

Byrne, J. (2010a) The Story of Relationship: Or coming to terms with my mother (and father). E-CENT Paper No.10. Hebden Bridge: The Institute for E-CENT. Available online: http://www.abc-counselling.com/id213.html

Byrne, J. (2010b) Self-acceptance and other-acceptance in relation to competence and morality. E-CENT Paper No.2(c). Hebden Bridge: The Institute for E-CENT. Available online: https://ecent-institute.org/e-cent-articles-and-papers/

Byrne, J. (2011) Completing your experience of difficult events, perceptions and painful emotions. E-CENT Paper No.13. Hebden Bridge: The Institute for Emotive-Cognitive Embodied Narrative Therapy. Available online: https://ecent-institute.org/e-cent-articles-and-papers/

Byrne, J. (2017) *Unfit for Therapeutic Purposes: The case against REBT/CBT.* Hebden Bridge: The Institute for E-CENT Publications.

Byrne, J. (2018a) *Lifestyle Counselling and Coaching for the Whole Person: Or how to integrate nutritional insights, exercise and sleep coaching into talk therapy*. Hebden Bridge: The Institute for E-CENT Publications.

Byrne, J. (2018b) *Top secrets for Building a Successful Relationship: Volume 1 – A blueprint and toolbox for couples and counsellors: C101*. Hebden Bridge: The Institute for E-CENT Publications.

Byrne, J. (2019) *Facing and Defeating your Emotional Dragons: How to process old traumas, and eliminate undigested pain from your past experience*. Hebden Bridge: The Institute for E-CENT Publications.

Cardwell, M. (2000) *The Complete A-Z Psychology Handbook*. Second edition. London: Hodder and Stoughton.

Carroll, H. (2016) 'How-losing-sleep-turns-women-MONSTERS'. *Daily Mail*: 13 January 2016. Available online: http://www.dailymail.co.uk/femail/article-3398358/ Date accessed: 5th June 2018.

Clinard, H.H. (1985) *Winning Ways to Succeed with People*. Houston: Gulf Publishing Company.

Campbell, T. (2014) Are smoothies good or bad? Newsletter, Centre for Nutrition Studies. Available online: http://nutritionstudies.org/are-smoothies-good-or-bad/. Accessed: 16th October 2017.

Cannon, W. (1927) The James-Lange theory of emotion: a critical examination and an alternative theory. *The American Journal of Psychology:* http://www.jstor.org/pss/1415404. Accessed: 15th March 2011.

Chaitow, L. (2003) *Candida Albicans: The non-drug approach to the treatment of Candida infection*. London: Thorsons.

Cherry, K. (2011) What is the Cannon-Bard theory? Online: http://psychology.about.com/ od/ cindex/g/cannonbard.htm. Accessed: 15th March 2011.

Clinard, H.H. (1985) *Winning Ways to Succeed with People*. Houston, TX: Gulf Publishing Inc.

Collins, N.L. and Read, S.J. (1990) Adult attachment, working models and relationship quality in dating couples. *Journal of Personality and Social Psychology 58:* 633-644.

Colman, A. (2002) *Dictionary of Psychology*. Oxford: Oxford University Press.

Cooper, J. and P.F. Procoupé (eds.) (1995) On Anger. In *Seneca*: *Moral and Political Essays*. (Trans. John Cooper and P.F. Procoupé). Cambridge: Cambridge University Press.

Cunningham, J. B. (2001) *The Stress Management Sourcebook. Second edition*. Los Angeles: Lowell House.

Damasio, A.R. (1994) *Descartes' Error: Emotion, Reason, and the Human Brain*. New York; Putnam.

Damasio, A.R. (2000) *The Feeling of What Happens: body, emotion and the making of consciousness*. London: Vintage.

Darwin, C. (1872/1965) *The Expression of the Emotions in Man and Animals*. Chicago: University of Chicago Press.

Darwin, C. (1898) *The Expression of the Emotions in Man and Animals.* New York: D. Appleton and Company. Page 237. Online at: Electronic Text Center, University of Virginia Library. Url: http://etext.virginia.edu/toc/modeng/public/ DarExpr.html. Accessed: 19th April 2011.

Dean, B. (2005) 'Forgiveness'. A positive psychology newsletter. Personal communication by email. No known online or paperback source.

Doidge, N. (2008) *The Brain that Changes Itself: Stories of personal triumph from the frontiers of brain science*. London: Penguin.

Edelman, S. (2006) *Change Your Thinking: overcome stress, combat anxiety and improve your life with CBT*. London: Vermillion.

Ekman, P. (1993) Facial expression and emotion. *American Psychologist 48 (4):* Pages 384-392.

Ellis, A. (1958). Rational Psychotherapy, *Journal of General Psychology,* 59, 35-49.

Ellis, A. (1962) *Reason and Emotion in Psychotherapy*. New York: Carol Publishing.

Epictetus (1991) *Enchiridion.* Trans. by George Long. New York: Prometheus Books.

Erwin, E. (1997) *Philosophy and Psychotherapy: Razing the troubles of the brain*, London, Sage.

Evans, D. (2003) *Emotion: a very short introduction.* Oxford. Oxford University Press.

Eysenck, M.W. and Keane, M.T. (2000) *Cognitive Psychology: A student's handbook.* Fourth edition. Philadelphia, PA: Psychology Press.

Fisher, M. (2005) *Beating Anger: The eight-point plan for coping with rage.* London: Rider.

Fonagy, P. (2001) *Attachment Theory and Psychoanalysis.* New York: Other Press.

Fonagy, P., Gergeley, G., Jurist, E.J., and Target, M.I. (2002) *Affect regulation, mentalization, and the development of the self.* New York: Other Press.

Freud, S. (1993) *Historical and Expository Works on Psychoanalysis. Volume 15.* London: Penguin Books.

Freud, S. (1995) Beyond the pleasure principle. In: Gay, P. (ed) *The Freud Reader.* London: Vintage Books.

Gerhardt, S. (2004) *Why Love Matters: How affection shapes a baby's brain.* London: Routledge.

Gesch, C.B., Hammond, S.M., Hampson, S.E., et.al. (2002) Influence of supplementary vitamins, minerals and essential fatty acids on the antisocial behaviour of young adult prisoners. Randomised, placebo-controlled trial. *British Journal of Psychiatry 181.* Pages 22-8.

Golomb, B.A., Evans, M.A., White, H.L., and Dimsdale, J.E. (2012) Trans-fat consumption and aggression. Online: PLoS One. 2012; 7(3):e32175. doi: 10.1371/journal.pone.0032175. Epub 2012 Mar 5.

Gordon, A.M. (2013) Up all night: The effects of sleep loss on mood. Research shows just one bad night of sleep can put a damper on your mood. *Psychology Today Online.* August 15th 2013. Available here: https://www.psychology today.com/ blog/ between-you-and-me/201308/all-night-the-effects-sleep-loss-mood. Accessed: 20th January 2018.

Griffin, J. and Tyrrell, I. (2004) *Human Givens: A new approach to emotional health and clear thinking.* Chalvington, East Sussex: HG Publishing.

Hartley, M. (2002) *Managing Anger at Work.* London: Sheldon Press.

Hazan, C. and Shaver P. (1990) Love and work: An attachment theoretical perspective. *Journal of Personality and Social Psychology 59:* 270-280.

Heller, S. (1998). 'Emerging field of forgiveness studies explores how we let go of grudges. *The Chronicle of Higher Education, July 17th 1998*.

Hobson, R.F. (1985) *Forms of Feeling: The heart of psychotherapy.* London: Routledge.

Holford, P. (2010) *Optimum Nutrition for the Mind*. London: Piatkus.

Iacoboni, M. (2008) *Mirroring People: The new science of how we connect with others.* New York: Farrar.

Irvine, W.B. (2009) *A Guide to the Good Life: The ancient art of Stoic joy*. Oxford: Oxford University Press.

Jacobs, E. (1994) *Impact Therapy*. Lutz, LF: Psychological Assessment Resources.

Jacobs, G. (1994) *Candida Albicans: A user's guide to treatment and recovery*. London: Optima.

Kagan, J. and Segal, J. (1992) *Psychology: An introduction.* Seventh edition. Fort Worth: Harcourt, Brace, Jovanovich College Publishers.

Keown, D. (2005) *Buddhist Ethics: A very short introduction*. Oxford: Oxford University Press.

Khoddam, R. (2014) 'The Psychology of Forgiveness: A how-to guide on the science behind learning to forgive'. Blog post on *Psychology Today*. Posted September 16th 2014, here: https://www.psychologytoday.com/us/blog/the-addiction-connection/201409/the-psychology-forgiveness. Accessed: 16th December 2018.

Kobak, R. and Sceery, A. (1988) Attachment in late adolescence working models, affect regulation and perceptions of self and others. *Child Development 59:* 135-146.

Kornfield, J. (1994) *Buddha's Little Instruction Book*. New York: Bantam Books.

Kornfield, J. (2002) *The Art of Forgiveness, Lovingkindness, and Peace*. London: Rider.

Lazarus, R.S. (1991). Progress on a cognitive-motivational-relational theory of Emotion. *American Psychologist, 46(8),* Pages 819-834.

Le Doux, J. (1996). *The Emotional Brain: the mysterious underpinnings of emotional life.* New York: Simon and Schuster.

Lewis, M. (2010) The development of anger. In: Potegal, N., Stemmler, G. and Spielberger, C. (eds) (2010) *International Handbook of Anger: Constituent and concomitant Biological, Psychological and Social processes*. New York: Springer.

Lewis, T., Amini, F. and Lannon, R. (2001) *A General Theory of Love*. New York: Vintage Books.

Lindenfield, G. (2000) *Managing Anger: Simple steps to dealing with frustration and threat.* London: Thorsons.

Lorenz, K. (1966/2002) *On Aggression.* London: Routledge.

Macaskill, A. (2002) Heal the Hurt: How to forgive and move on. London: Sheldon Press.

Mascaró, J. (1973/2015) *The Dhammapada.* London: Penguin Books (Little Black Classics No.80).

Mehrabian, A. (1981) *Silent Messages: Implicit communication of emotions and attitudes.* Belmont, CA: Wadsworth (currently distributed by Albert Mehrabian, email: am@kaaj.com)

Mosley, M. (2015) 'Which oils are best to cook with?' 28th July 2015. *BBC: News: Magazine*, 28th July 2015. Online: http://www.bbc.co.uk/news/magazine-33675975

My-Sahana (2012) Common Causes for Anger Management Issues. MySahana blog post. Online: http://mysahana.org/2012/02/common-causes-for-anger-manage-ment-issues/. Accessed: 22nd January 2018.

O'Brien, B. (2011) Anger and Buddhism: What Buddhism Teaches About Anger. Available online: http://buddhism.about.com/od/basicbuddhistteachings/a/ anger. htm. Accessed: 14th March 2011.

Panksepp, J. (1998) *Affective Neuroscience: The foundations of human and animal emotions.* Oxford University Press.

Panksepp, J. and Lucy Biven (2012) *The Archaeology of Mind: Neuroevolutionary Origins of Human Emotion*: W.W. Norton and Company. See the book description here: http://www.amazon.co.uk/The-Archaeology-Mind-Neuroevolutionary-Interpersonal/dp/0393705315

Perretta, L. (2001) *Brain Food: the essential guide to boosting brain power.* London: Hamlyn.

Peterson, C., & Seligman, M. E. P. (2004). *Character strengths and virtues: A handbook and classification.* Washington, DC: American Psychological Association.

Philpot, C. (2006). Intergroup apologies and forgiveness. Unpublished PhD thesis, University of Queensland, Brisbane, Australia. Online: https://www.scribd .com/document/328941790/forgiveness-pdf. Accessed: 30th November 2018.

Pinker, S. (2015) *How the Mind Works.* London: Penguin Random House.

Potegal, M. and Novoco, R.W. (2010) A brief history of anger. In: Potegal, N., Stemmler, G. and Spielberger, C. (eds) (2010) *International Handbook of Anger: Constituent and concomitant Biological, Psychological and Social processes*. New York: Springer.

Potegal, M. and Stemmler, G. (2010) Cross-disciplinary view of anger: consensus and controversy. In: Potegal, N., Stemmler, G. and Spielberger, C. (eds) (2010) *International Handbook of Anger: Constituent and concomitant Biological, Psychological and Social processes*. New York: Springer.

Ratcliffe, S. (ed) (2010) *Oxford Dictionary of Quotations, Second edition*. Oxford: Oxford University Press.

Reynolds, G. (2010) Phys Ed: Can Exercise Moderate Anger? August 11, 2010. Available online, here: http://well.blogs.nytimes.com/2010/08/11/phys-ed-can-exercise-moderate-anger/?_r=0. Accessed: 16th June 2016.

Robinson, P. (2011) 'Could I send Mr Angry packing?' An article in the Femail section of the *Daily Mail Online*. 28th April 2011. Available online on this url: http://www.dailymail.co.uk/femail/article-1380989/Could-I-send-Mr-Angry-Packing-Horrified-repeatedly-raging-children-Philip-Robinson-tried-unconventional-therapy.html. Accessed: 6th June 2011.

Ross, J. (2002) *The Mood Cure: Take charge of your emotions in 24 hours using food and supplements.* London: Thorsons.

Satir, V. (1972/1983) *Peoplemaking*. London: Souvenir Press.

Schoenthaler, S.J. (1983) 'The Northern California diet-behaviour program: An empirical evaluation of 3,000 incarcerated juveniles in Stanislaus County Juvenile Hall'. *International Journal of Biosocial Research, Vol 5(2),* Pages 99-106.

Schoenthaler, S.J. (1983) 'The Los Angeles probation department diet behaviour program: An empirical analysis of six institutional settings'. *International Journal of Biosocial Research, Vol 5(2),* Pages 107-117.

Schoenthaler S., et al (1997) 'The effect of randomized vitamin-mineral supplementation on violent and non-violent antisocial behaviour among incarcerated juveniles'. *Journal of Nutritional & Environmental Medicine 7:* Pages 343–352.

Schoenthaler, S., and Bier I. D. (2002) 'Food addiction and criminal behaviour – The California randomized trial'. *Food Allergy and Intolerance. 731–746.*

Schore, A. N. (2003) *Affect regulation and the repair of the self.* New York: Norton.

Schore, A.N. (2015) *Affect Regulation and the Origin of the Self: The Neurobiology of Emotional Development*. London: Routledge.

Seddon, K. (2000) The Stoics on why we should strive to be free of the passions. *Practical Philosophy, Vol.3:3,* November 2000. Available online: http://www.wku.edu/ ~jan.garrett/stoa/seddon2.htm. Accessed: 14th March 2011.

Siegel, D.J. (2015) *The Developing Mind: How relationships and the brain interact to shape who we are.* London: The Guilford Press.

Simopoulos, A.P. (2002) 'The importance of the ratio of omega-6/omega-3 essential fatty acids'. *Biomedical Pharmacotherapy, Oct 2002, Vol. 56 (8):* Pages 365-379.

Simpson, J.A., Rholes, W.S., and Nelligan, J.S. (1992) Support seeking and support giving within couples in an anxiety provoking situation: The role of attachment styles. *Journal of Personality and Social Psychology 60:* 434-446.

Sloane, W. (2010) *Anger Management: The essential guide.* Peterborough, UK: Need2Know/Forward Press Limited.

Smith, A. (1984) *The Mind.* London: Hodder and Stoughton.

Smith, P.K., Cowie, H., and Blades, M. (2011) *Understanding Children's Development. Fifth edition.* Chichester, West Sussex: Wiley.

Soanes, C. (2002) *Paperback Oxford English Dictionary.* New York: Oxford University Press.

Sonkin, D. (2011) Anger: Attachment and neurobiological perspectives. Blog: Available online: http://daniel.sonkin .com/anger-attachment.html. Accessed: 15th March 2011.

Sri Rahula, W. (1997) *What the Buddha Taught.* Oxford: Oneworld Publications.

Steiner, C. (1997) *Achieving Emotional Literacy: A personal program to increase you emotional intelligence.* London: Bloomsbury.

Stress Management Society (2012/2016) Nutritional stress and health: The "Think 'nervous'" box. Available online: http://www.stress.org.uk/Diet-and-nutrition.aspx

Suzuki, S. (1999) *Zen Mind, Beginner's Mind.* New York: Weatherhill.

Taylor-Byrne, R.E., and Byrne, J.W. (2017) *How to Control Your Anger, Anxiety and Depression, Using nutrition and physical activity.* Hebden Bridge: The Institute for E-CENT Publications.

Taylor-Byrne, R.E. (In press) *Safeguard Your Sleep and Reap the Rewards: Better health, happiness and resilience*. Hebden Bridge: The Institute for E-CENT Publications.

The Real Food Guide (2017) 'What is margarine and why is it bad for you?' An online blog: http://therealfoodguide.com/what-is-margarine-and-why-is-it-bad-for-you/

Tkacz, J., et al. (2008) Aerobic exercise program reduces anger expression among overweight children. Paediatric Exercise Science, 2008 Nov; Vol.20 (4): Pages 390-401.

Trowbridge, J.P. and Walker, M. (1989) *The Yeast Syndrome*. London: Bantam Books.

Turner, J.H. (2000) *On the Origins of Human Emotions. A sociological inquiry into the evolution of human affect.* Stanford University Press. See the book outline at this website: http://www.sup.org/ books/title/?id=436

Vaillant, G.E. (1992) *Ego Mechanisms of Defence: A guide for clinicians and researchers.* Washington DC: American Psychiatric Association Press.

Vitelli, R. (2016) 'Does Lack of Sleep Make People More Violent?' Available online: https://www.psychologytoday .com/gb/blog/media-spotlight/201610/does-lack-sleep-make-people-more-violent. Date accessed 8th June 2018.

Walker, M. (2017) *Why We Sleep*. London: Allen Lane.

Wallin, D. (2007) *Attachment in Psychotherapy.* New York: The Guildford Press.

Watts, A. (1962/1990) *The Way of Zen.* London: Arkana/Penguin.

Winston, R. (2003) *The Human Mind: And how to make the most of it.* London: Bantam Books.

Wood, D. (1988) *How Children Think and Learn.* Oxford: Blackwell.

Woodward, N. (2006) Stress, Diet and Body Acidification. Listed in *Cellular Chemistry*, originally published in issue 130 - December 2006. Available online at: http://www.positivehealth.com/ article/ alkaline/stress-diet- and-body-acidification

Yu, W. (2012) High trans-fat diet predicts aggression: People who eat more hydrogenated oils are more aggressive. *Scientific American Mind*, July 2012. Available online: http://www.scientificamerican.com/article/high-trans-fat-diet-predicts-aggresion/

Zimbardo, P. G., Banks, W.C., Craig, H. and Jaffe, D. (1973) A Pirandellian prison: The mind is a formidable jailor. *New York Times Magazine, April 8th,* 38-60.

Zimbardo, P. (2007) *The Lucifer Effect: how good people turn evil.* London: Rider.

~~~

Get your anger under reasonable control

Endnotes

[1] Byrne, J. (2009a) A journey through models of mind. The story of my personal origins. E-CENT Paper No.4. Hebden Bridge: The Institute for E-CENT.

[2] Byrne, J. (2010a) The Story of Relationship: Or coming to terms with my mother (and father). E-CENT Paper No.10. Hebden Bridge: The Institute for E-CENT. Available online: http://www.abc-counselling.com/id213.html

[3] Alan Paton quote, from page 198 of this book:

Ratcliffe, S. (ed) (2010) *Oxford Dictionary of Quotations, Second edition*. Oxford: Oxford University Press.

[4] Soanes, C. (2002) *Paperback Oxford English Dictionary.* New York: Oxford University Press.

[5] Colman, A. (2002) *Dictionary of Psychology*. Oxford: Oxford University Press.

[6] Khoddam, R. (2014) 'The Psychology of Forgiveness: A how-to guide on the science behind learning to forgive'. Blog post on *Psychology Today*. Posted September 16th 2014, here: https://www.psychologytoday.com/us/blog/the-addiction-connection/201409/the-psychology-forgiveness. Accessed: 16th December 2018.

[7] APA (2006) 'Forgiveness—Definitions and Effects'. Adapted from Philpot, C. (2006). Intergroup apologies and forgiveness. Unpublished PhD thesis, University of Queensland, Brisbane, Australia. Online: https://www.scribd .com/document/328941790/forgiveness-pdf. Accessed: 30th November 2018.

[8] Dean, B. (2005) 'Forgiveness'. A positive psychology newsletter. Personal communication by email. No known online or paperback source.

[9] Baskin and Enright (2004). 'Intervention studies on forgiveness: A meta-analysis.' *Journal of Counseling and Development 82*, 79-90.

[10] Blackburn, S. (1996) *Dictionary of Philosophy*. Oxford: Oxford University Press.

[11] Ratcliffe, S. (ed) (2010) *Oxford Dictionary of Quotations, Second edition*. Oxford: Oxford University Press. Page 197.

[12] Peterson, C., & Seligman, M. E. P. (2004). *Character strengths and virtues: A handbook and classification*. Washington, DC: American Psychological Association.

[13] Kornfield, J. (2002) *The Art of Forgiveness, Lovingkindness, and Peace*. London: Rider.

[14] Heller, S. (1998). 'Emerging field of forgiveness studies explores how we let go of grudges. *The Chronicle of Higher Education, July 17th 1998.*

[15] Soanes, C. (2002) *Paperback Oxford English Dictionary.* New York: Oxford University Press.

[16] Colman, A. (2002) *Dictionary of Psychology.* Oxford: Oxford University Press.

[17] Edelman, S. (2006) *Change Your Thinking: overcome stress, combat anxiety and improve your life with CBT.* London: Vermillion.

[18] Soanes, C. (2002) *Paperback Oxford English Dictionary.* New York: Oxford University Press.

[19] Fisher, M. (2005) *Beating Anger: The eight-point plan for coping with rage.* London: Rider.

[20] Darwin, C. (1898) *The Expression of the Emotions in Man and Animals.* New York: D. Appleton and Company. Page 237. Online at: Electronic Text Center, University of Virginia Library. Url: http://etext.virginia.edu/toc/modeng/public/ DarExpr.html. Accessed: 19th April 2011.

[21] Potegal, M. and Novoco, R.W. (2010) A brief history of anger. In: Potegal, N., Stemmler, G. and Spielberger, C. (eds) (2010) *International Handbook of Anger: Constituent and concomitant Biological, Psychological and Social processes.* New York: Springer.

[22] Lewis, M. (2010) The development of anger. In: Potegal, N., Stemmler, G. and Spielberger, C. (eds) (2010) *International Handbook of Anger: Constituent and concomitant Biological, Psychological and Social processes.* New York: Springer.

[23] Potegal, M. and Stemmler, G. (2010) Cross-disciplinary view of anger: consensus and controversy. In: Potegal, N., Stemmler, G. and Spielberger, C. (eds) (2010) *International Handbook of Anger: Constituent and concomitant Biological, Psychological and Social processes.* New York: Springer.

[24] Fisher (2005), pages 24-28.

[25] Griffin, J. and Tyrrell, I. (2004) *Human Givens: A new approach to emotional health and clear thinking.* Chalvington, East Sussex: HG Publishing. And Fisher (2005), page 32.

[26] Hartley, M. (2002) *Managing Anger at Work.* London: Sheldon Press. Page 1-2.

[27] Smith, A. (1984) The Mind. London: Hodder and Stoughton.

[28] Eysenck, M.W. and Keane, M.T. (2000) *Cognitive Psychology: a student's handbook.* Fourth edition. Philadelphia, PA: Psychology Press.

[29] Kagan, J. and Segal, J. (1992) *Psychology: an introduction.* Seventh edition. Fort Worth: Harcourt, Brace, Jovanovich College Publishers.

[30] Cannon, W. (1927) The James-Lange theory of emotion: a critical examination and an alternative theory. *The American Journal of Psychology:* http://www.jstor.org/pss/1415404. Accessed: 15th March 2011.

[31] Le Doux, J. (1996). *The Emotional Brain: the mysterious underpinnings of emotional life.* New York: Simon and Schuster.

[32] Damasio, A.R. (1994) Descartes' Error: Emotion, Reason, and the Human Brain. New York; Putnam. And:

Damasio, A.R. (2000) *The Feeling of What Happens: body, emotion and the making of consciousness.* London: Vintage.

[33] Cherry, K. (2011) What is the Cannon-Bard theory? Online: http://psychology.about.com/od/cindex/g/cannonbard.htm. Accessed: 15th March 2011.

[34] Lazarus, R.S. (1991). Progress on a cognitive-motivational-relational theory of Emotion. *American Psychologist, 46(8),* Pages 819-834.

[35] Byrne, J. (2017) *Unfit for Therapeutic Purposes: The case against REBT/CBT.* Hebden Bridge: The Institute for E-CENT Publications.

[36] Winston, R. (2003) *The Human Mind: and how to make the most of it.* London: Bantam Books.

[37] Lorenz, K. (1966/2002) *On Aggression.* London: Routledge.

[38] Freud, S. (1995) Beyond the pleasure principle. In: Gay, P. (ed) *The Freud Reader.* London: Vintage Books. Pages 594-595; 618-621.

[39] Freud, S. (1993) *Historical and Expository Works on Psychoanalysis. Volume15.* London: Penguin Books.

[40]   . Found on The Free Dictionary, by Farlex (Online): at: http://medical-dictionary.thefree dictionary.com/constructive+aggression. Accessed: 8th April 2011.

[41] Aggression /ag·gres·sion/ (ah-gresh´un) Behaviour leading to self-assertion; it may arise from innate drives and/or a response to frustration, and may be manifested by destructive and attacking behaviour, by hostility and obstructionism, or by self-expressive drive to mastery. Source: Dorland's Medical Dictionary for Health Consumers. © 2007 by Saunders, an imprint of Elsevier, Inc. Found here: http://medical-dictionary.thefreedictionary.com/aggression. Accessed: 8th April 2011.

[42] Lorenz, K. (1966/2002) *On Aggression.* London: Routledge.

[43] Bandura, A., Ross, D., and Ross, S.A. (1961) Transmission of aggression through imitation of aggressive models. *Journal of Abnormal and Social Psychology, 63,* Pages 572-582.

[44] Banyard, P. and Grayson, A. (2000) *Introducing Psychological Research: Seventy studies that shape psychology*. Second edition. Basingstoke, Hampshire: Palgrave.

[45] Hartley, M. (2002) *Managing Anger at Work.* London: Sheldon Press. Page 3.

[46] Zimbardo, P. G., Banks, W.C., Craig, H. and Jaffe, D. (1973) A Pirandellian prison: The mind is a formidable jailor. *New York Times Magazine, April 8th,* 38-60. And:

Zimbardo, P. (2007) *The Lucifer Effect: how good people turn evil.* London: Rider.

[47] Hartley, M. (2002) *Managing Anger at Work.* London: Sheldon Press. Pages 4-5.

[48] Bowlby, J. (1988/2005) *A Secure Base: clinical applications of attachment theory.* London: Routledge Classics.

[49] Sonkin, D. (2011) Anger: Attachment and neurobiological perspectives. Available online: http://daniel.sonkin.com/anger-attachment.html. Accessed: 15th March 2011.

[50] Bowlby, J. (1988/2005)

[51] Lewis, T., Amini, F. and Lannon, R. (2001) *A General Theory of Love.* New York: Vintage Books.

[52] Gerhardt, S. (2004) *Why Love Matters: How affection shapes a baby's brain.* London: Routledge.

[53] Wallin, D. (2007) *Attachment in Psychotherapy.* New York: The Guildford Press.

[54] Fonagy, P., Gergeley, G., Jurist, E.J., and Target, M.I. (2002) *Affect regulation, mentalization, and the development of the self.* New York: Other Press.

[55] Schore, A. N. (2003) Affect regulation and the repair of the self. New York: Norton.

[56] Fonagy, P. (2001) *Attachment Theory and Psychoanalysis*. New York: Other Press.

[57] Collins, N.L. and Read, S.J. (1990) Adult attachment, working models and relationship quality in dating couples. *Journal of Personality and Social Psychology 58:* 633-644.

[58] Kobak, R. and Sceery, A. (1988) Attachment in late adolescence working models, affect regulation and perceptions of self and others. *Child Development 59:* 135-146.

[59] Simpson, J.A., Rholes, W.S., and Nelligan, J.S. (1992) Support seeking and support giving within couples in an anxiety provoking situation: the role of attachment styles. *Journal of Personality and Social Psychology 60:* 434-446.

[60] Vaillant, G.E. (1992) *Ego Mechanisms of Defence: A guide for clinicians and researchers.* Washington DC: American Psychiatric Association Press.

[61] Armsden, G.C. and Greenberg, M.T. (1987) The inventory of parent and peer attachment: individual differences and their relationship to psychological well-being in adolescence. *Journal of Youth and Adolescence 16:* 427-454.

[62] Hazan, C. and Shaver P. (1990) Love and work: an attachment theoretical perspective. *Journal of Personality and Social Psychology 59:* 270-280.

[63] "(The) *Dismissing* (type of) adults appear to be relatively resistant to treatment and within the context of therapy. Arguably, they deny their need for help in order to protect themselves from the possibility that the caregiver will be eventually unavailable. They might be rejecting of treatment, rarely asking for help (Dozier 1990)". Quoted from Fonagy, 2001, page 34.

[64] "(The) *Preoccupied* (type of) adults have a more general inability to collaborate with and take in the therapist's words and support, but then become dependent and call therapists between hours (Dozier et al 1991)". Quoted from Fonagy 2001, page 34.

[65] Fonagy (2001) presents a new way of conceptualizing the work of the attachment theorists: "A synthetic view of this literature has been suggested by Sidney Blatt and colleagues (Blatt and Blass 1996, Blatt et al 1995, Blatt et al 1998). Blatt and his co-workers have proposed a dichotomy that overlaps in a highly informative way with the Bowlby-Ainsworth-main categorization (of attachment styles). They envision a dialectic between two developmental pressures that defines the evolving representations of self-other relationships: the needs for a sense of relatedness and a sense of autonomous identity (Blatt and Blass 1996). These developmental needs are thought to be in synergistic interaction throughout (childhood development) and a lack of balance implies psychopathology". Quoted from Fonagy (2001), page 34.

[66] Doidge, N. (2008) *The Brain that Changes Itself: stories of personal triumph from the frontiers of brain science.* London: Penguin.

[6767] Visceral reactions refer to deep body feelings, as opposed to feelings (affects) in the mind.

[68] Griffin, J. and Tyrrell, I. (2004) *Human Givens: A new approach to emotional health and clear thinking.* Chalvington, East Sussex: HG Publishing.

[69] Seneca (1995) On anger. In *Moral and Political Essays.* Trans. John Cooper and P.F. Procoupé. Cambridge: Cambridge University Press.

[70] Aurelius, Marcus (1992. *Meditations.* Trans. by A.S.L. Farquharson. London: Everyman's Library.

[71] Epictetus (1991) *Enchiridion.* Trans. by George Long. New York: Prometheus Books.

[72] Irvine, W.B. (2009) *A Guide to the Good Life: The ancient art of Stoic joy.* Oxford: Oxford University Press.

[73] BCE = BC in the Christian system of dating events before or after Christ.

[74] Seddon, K. (2000) The Stoics on why we should strive to be free of the passions. *Practical Philosophy, Vol.3:3,* November 2000. Available online: http://www.wku.edu/ ~jan.garrett/stoa/seddon2.htm. Accessed: 14th March 2011.

[75] The concept of 'Opinions' here means 'perceptions, judgements, and evaluations'.

[76] Of course, when I say "it should be the way it is", I am excluding "moral shoulds". It could be that somebody "morally should not have struck you" – but if s/he did, then s/he did, and it does not make sense to say s/he "absolutely (in a non-moral sense) should not have done what she did". It was morally wrong, and it would have been **preferable** if s/he had not done it. (And she should be taught to refrain from such bad act, to the extent that is possible to teach her anything). But there is no law of the universe that says: "When something is immoral, it ABSOLUTELY must not happen!" We have moral rules precisely because immoral acts DO ACTUALLY HAPPEN!

[77] Byrne, J. with Renata Taylor-Byrne (2018) *Lifestyle Counselling and Coaching for the Whole Person: Or how to integrate nutritional insights, exercise and sleep coaching into talk therapy*. Hebden Bridge: The Institute for E-CENT Publications.

[78] Irvine, W.B. (2009) *A Guide to the Good Life: the ancient art of Stoic joy*. Oxford: Oxford University Press. Chapter 6.

[79] Ben-Shahar, T. (2007) *Happier: Learn the secrets to daily joy and lasting fulfilment*. New York: McGraw-Hill.

[80] Page 41: Epictetus (1991) *Enchiridion*. Trans. by George Long. New York: Prometheus Books.

[81] Jacobs, E. (1994) *Impact Therapy*. Lutz, LF: Psychological Assessment Resources.

[82] Aurelius, M. (1992). *Meditations*. Trans. by A.S.L. Farquharson. London: Everyman's Library. Book II: page 7.

[83] Sri Rahula, W. (1997) *What the Buddha Taught*. Oxford: Oneworld Publications. Page 16.

[84] Or, as Alan Watts puts it: "The point is rather that life as we usually live it is suffering – or, more exactly, is bedevilled by the peculiar frustration which comes from attempting the impossible. Perhaps, then, 'frustration' is the best equivalent for *dukkha*..." even though the word is the opposite of 'pleasant' or 'sweet' – making it mean "unpleasant" or "bitter". (Watts, A. (1962/1990) *The Way of Zen*. London: Arkana/Penguin. Page 66)

[85] And Watts (1962/1990) renders the cause of frustration as 'trishna', which he translates as "...clinging or grasping, based on *avidya*, which is ignorance or unconsciousness. (Watts, page 67)

[86] "It is this 'thirst', desire, greed, craving, manifesting itself in various ways, that gives rise to all forms of suffering …". Page 29, Sri Rahula (1997).

[87] Keown, D. (2005) *Buddhist Ethics: a very short introduction.* Oxford: Oxford University Press.

[88] Kornfield, J. (1994) Buddha's Little Instruction Book. New York: Bantam Books.

[89] O'Brien, B. (2011) Anger and Buddhism: What Buddhism Teaches About Anger. Available online: http://buddhism.about.com/od/basicbuddhistteachings/ a/anger. htm. Accessed: 14th March 2011.

[90] Buddhism Online (2011) A view on Buddhism: Anger and Aversion. Available online: http://viewonbuddhism.org/anger.html. Accessed: 14th March 2011.

[91] Beck, C.J. (1997) *Everyday Zen: love and work.* London: Thorsons. Pages 53-61.

[92] Buddhism Online (2011) A view on Buddhism: Anger and Aversion. Available online: http://viewonbuddhism.org/anger.html. Accessed: 14th March 2011. Page 2.

[93] Or, more colourfully: "We are all bozos on the same bus". Sheldon Kopp.

[94] Cf: Suzuki, S. (1999) *Zen Mind, Beginner's Mind.* New York: Weatherhill.

[95] Steiner, C. (1997) *Achieving Emotional Literacy: A personal program to increase you emotional intelligence.* London: Bloomsbury.

[96] Clinard, H.H. (1985) *Winning Ways to Succeed with People.* Houston, TX: Gulf Publishing Inc.

[97] From: Buddhism Online (2011) A view on Buddhism: Anger and Aversion. Available online: http://viewonbuddhism.org/anger.html. Accessed: 14th March 2011. Pages 8-10.

[98] "Our brains are wired up to experience what others are experiencing". (Sonkin, 2011, page 8). And: Iacoboni, M. (2008) *Mirroring People: The new science of how we connect with others.* New York: Farrar.

[99] Ellis, A. (1962) *Reason and Emotion in Psychotherapy.* New York: Carol Publishing.

[100] Beck, A.T. (1976/1989). *Cognitive Therapy and the Emotional Disorders.* London: Penguin Books.

[101] Beck, A.T. (1999) *Prisoners of Hate: The Cognitive Basis of Anger, Hostility, and Violence*. New York: HarperCollins.

[102] Burns, D. (1990) *The Feeling Good Handbook.* New York: Penguin/Plume.

[103] Edelman, S. (2006) *Change Your Thinking: overcome stress, combat anxiety and improve your life with CBT.* London: Vermillion.

[104] I am pleased that Dr Sarah Edelman mentions exercise and relaxation. Relaxation has a secure existence in most systems of therapy which came out of behaviour therapy, or which were influenced by behaviour therapy. Physical exercise does not often get a mention, and it was not normally advocated by Albert Ellis or Aaron Tim Beck. Arnold Lazarus's Multimodal Therapy is probably the only behaviour-therapy derived system – and apart from E-CENT, probably the *only* system - that focuses significant attention on to diet, exercise and self-talk as a cluster of causative/curative elements in the aetiology/resolution of emotional disturbance. See in particular: Lazarus (1989), in the References at the end of this article.

[105] Bandura, A., Ross, D., and Ross, S.A. (1961) Transmission of aggression through imitation of aggressive models. *Journal of Abnormal and Social Psychology, 63,* Pages 572-582.

[106] Aurelius, M. (1991) *Meditations.* Trans. by A.S.L. Farquharson. London: Everyman's Library.

[107] Byrne, J. (2009b) The 'Individual' and his/her Social Relationships - The E-CENT Perspective. E-CENT Paper No. 9. Hebden Bridge: The Institute for E-CENT. Available online: https://ecent-institute.org/e-cent-articles-and-papers/.

[108] Griffin, J. and Tyrrell, I. (2004) *Human Givens: A new approach to emotional health and clear thinking.* Chalvington, East Sussex: HG Publishing.

[109] Byrne, J. (2010b) Self-acceptance and other-acceptance in relation to competence and morality. E-CENT Paper No.2(c). Hebden Bridge: The Institute for E-CENT. Available online: https://ecent-institute.org/e-cent-articles-and-papers/

[110] Here is the reference for a much later book by Chaitow: Chaitow, L. (2003) *Candida Albicans: The non-drug approach to the treatment of Candida infection.* London: Thorsons.

[111] Two additional sources on Candida Albicans and the link to physical illness and emotional distress:

Jacobs, G. (1994) *Candida Albicans: A user's guide to treatment and recovery*. London: Optima. And:

Trowbridge, J.P. and Walker, M. (1989) *The Yeast Syndrome*. London: Bantam Books.

[112] Golomb, B.A., Evans, M.A., White, H.L., and Dimsdale, J.E. (2012) Trans-fat consumption and aggression. Online: PLoS One. 2012; 7(3):e32175. doi: 10.1371/journal.pone.0032175. Epub 2012 Mar 5.

[113] **Definition** of Mediterranean diet: A diet of a type traditional in Mediterranean countries, characterized especially by a high consumption of vegetables and olive oil and moderate consumption of protein, and thought to confer health benefits.

[114] Definition of Paleo diet: A diet based on the types of foods presumed to have been eaten by early humans, consisting chiefly of meat, fish, vegetables, and fruit and excluding dairy or cereal products and processed food.

[115] Simopoulos (2002) produced a study which argues for a low ratio of omega-6 to omega-3 fatty acids. Here is the abstract from that paper:

"Abstract:

"Several sources of information suggest that human beings evolved on a diet with a ratio of omega-6 to omega-3 essential fatty acids (EFA) of approximately 1 whereas in Western diets the ratio is 15/1-16.7/1. Western diets are deficient in omega-3 fatty acids, and have excessive amounts of omega-6 fatty acids compared with the diet on which human beings evolved and their genetic patterns were established. Excessive amounts of omega-6 polyunsaturated fatty acids (PUFA) and a very high omega-6/omega-3 ratio, as is found in today's Western diets, promote the pathogenesis of many diseases, including cardiovascular disease, cancer, and inflammatory and autoimmune diseases, whereas increased levels of omega-3 PUFA (a low omega-6/omega-3 ratio) exert suppressive effects. In the secondary prevention of cardiovascular disease, a ratio of 4/1 was associated with a 70% decrease in total mortality. A ratio of 2.5/1 reduced rectal cell proliferation in patients with colorectal cancer, whereas a ratio of 4/1 with the same amount of omega-3 PUFA had no effect. The lower omega-6/omega-3 ratio in women with breast cancer was associated with decreased risk. A ratio of 2-3/1 suppressed inflammation in patients with rheumatoid arthritis, and a ratio of 5/1 had a beneficial effect on patients with asthma, whereas a ratio of 10/1 had adverse consequences. These studies indicate that the optimal ratio may vary with the disease under consideration.

This is consistent with the fact that chronic diseases are multigenic and multifactorial. Therefore, it is quite possible that the therapeutic dose of omega-3 fatty acids will depend on the degree of severity of disease resulting from the genetic predisposition. A lower ratio of omega-6/omega-3 fatty acids is more desirable in reducing the risk of many of the chronic diseases of high prevalence in Western societies, as well as in the developing countries, that are being exported to the rest of the world." Source: Simopoulos, A.P. (2002) 'The importance of the ratio of omega-6/omega-3 essential fatty acids'. *Biomedical Pharmacotherapy, Oct 2002, Vol.56 (8):* Pages 365-379.

~~~

[116] Cunningham, J. B. (2001) The Stress Management Sourcebook. Second edition. Los Angeles: Lowell House.

[117] Winnie Yu (2012) High trans-fat diet predicts aggression: People who eat more hydrogenated oils are more aggressive. *Scientific American Mind*, July 2012. Available online: http://www.scientificamerican.com/article/high-trans-fat-diet-predicts-aggresion/

[118] Stress Management Society (2012/2016) Nutritional stress and health: The "Think 'nervous'" box. Available online: http://www.stress.org.uk/Diet-and-nutrition.aspx

[119] "A diet high in refined carbohydrates may lead to an increased risk for new-onset depression in postmenopausal women, according to a study published in The American Journal of Clinical Nutrition.

"The study by James Gangwisch, PhD and colleagues in the department of psychiatry at Columbia University Medical Centre (CUMC) looked at the dietary glycaemic index, glycaemic load, types of carbohydrates consumed, and depression in data from more than 70,000 postmenopausal women who participated in the National Institutes of Health's Women's Health Initiative Observational Study between 1994 and 1998." Available online: https://www.sciencedaily. com/releases/2015/08/ 150805110335. htm. Accessed: 3rd October 2017.

~~~

[120] Perretta, Lorraine (2001) *Brain Food: the essential guide to boosting brain power.* London: Hamlyn.

[121] Cunningham, J. B. (2001) *The Stress Management Sourcebook.* Second edition. Los Angeles: Lowell House.

[122] Woodward, N. (2006) Stress, Diet and Body Acidification. Listed in *Cellular Chemistry*, originally published in issue 130 - December 2006. Available online at: http://www.positivehealth.com/article/alkaline/stress-diet- and-body-acidification

[123] The research on milk and the emotional and behavioural effects upon a group of children, in a double blind study, published in the Lancet in the UK, has been largely ignored by policy makers. Here is a flavour of the problem, from the opening of a blog by Dr H Morrow Brown MD, FRCP (Edin), FAAAAI (USA):

"The emotional aspects of milk intolerance are so variable and so bizarre that it is difficult to select the most interesting and illustrative cases seen over the years. Emotional effects along with gastro-intestinal symptoms are commonly associated with migraine. Milk intolerant children often have a short attention span, cannot sit still, and have tantrums and poor coordination. A tendency to self-injury and destructiveness sometimes occurs repeatedly after drinking milk. Their poor coordination is obvious in their writing and "art work", because meaningless squiggles become recognizable objects or people after withdrawal of the relevant foods."

We believe it is important, because of this research, to limit the amount of dairy milk that we consume, and to substitute nut or rice milk where possible.

~~~

[124] Source: Campbell, T. (2014) Are smoothies good or bad? Newsletter, Centre for Nutrition Studies. Available online: http://nutritionstudies.org/are-smoothies-good-or-bad/. Accessed: 16th October 2017.

[125] Source: The Real Food Guide (2017) 'What is margarine and why is it bad for you?' An online blog: http://therealfoodguide.com/what-is-margarine-and-why-is-it-bad-for-you/

[126] Mosley, M. (2015) 'Which oils are best to cook with?' 28th July 2015. BBC: News: Magazine, 28th July 2015. Online: http://www.bbc.co.uk/news/magazine-33675975

[127] Dr John Briffa, 'High Anxiety', *Observer Magazine,* 19th June 2005, page 61.

[128] Perretta, L. (2001) *Brain Food: the essential guide to boosting brain power.* London: Hamlyn.

[129] Lettuce and anxiety are mentioned in this blog: http://www.organicfacts.net/health-benefits/vegetable/health-benefits-of-lettuce.html

[130] Chamomile tea for anxiety and insomnia; mentioned in this blog: http://naturalsociety.com/9-amazing-health-benefits-of-chamomile-tea/

[131] Blog address for Health Unblocked post about Chamomile tea and SSRI's: https://healthunlocked.com/anxietysupport/posts/132860526/can-camomile-tea-interfere-with-anti-depressants-and-antibiotics

[132] Byrne, J. with Renata Taylor-Byrne (2018) *Lifestyle Counselling and Coaching for the Whole Person: Or how to integrate nutritional insights, exercise and sleep coaching into talk therapy.* Hebden Bridge: The Institute for E-CENT Publications.

[133] Taylor-Byrne, R.E., and Byrne, J.W. (2017) *How to Control Your Anger, Anxiety and Depression, Using nutrition and physical activity.* Hebden Bridge: The Institute for E-CENT Publications.

[134] Ross, J. (2002) *The Mood Cure: Take charge of your emotions in 24 hours using food and supplements.* London: Thorsons.

[135] Holford, P. (2010) *Optimum Nutrition for the Mind.* London: Piatkus.

[136] Schoenthaler, S.J. (1983) 'The Northern California diet-behaviour program: An empirical evaluation of 3,000 incarcerated juveniles in Stanislaus County Juvenile Hall'. *International Journal of Biosocial Research, Vol 5(2),* Pages 99-106.

Schoenthaler, S.J. (1983) 'The Los Angeles probation department diet behaviour program: An empirical analysis of six institutional settings'. *International Journal of Biosocial Research, Vol 5(2),* Pages 107-117.

Schoenthaler S., et al (1997) 'The effect of randomized vitamin-mineral supplementation on violent and non-violent antisocial behaviour among incarcerated juveniles'. *Journal of Nutritional & Environmental Medicine 7:* Pages 343–352.

Schoenthaler, S., and Bier I. D. (2002) 'Food addiction and criminal behaviour – The California randomized trial'. *Food Allergy and Intolerance. 731–746.* Saunders. Cited in Sandwell and Wheatley (2008).

~~~

[137] Gesch, C.B., Hammond, S.M., Hampson, S.E., et.al. (2002) Influence of supplementary vitamins, minerals and essential fatty acids on the antisocial behaviour of young adult prisoners. Randomised, placebo-controlled trial. *British Journal of Psychiatry 181.* Pages 22-8.

[138] Tkacz, J., et al. (2008) Aerobic exercise program reduces anger expression among overweight children. Paediatric Exercise Science, 2008 Nov; Vol.20 (4): Pages 390-401.

[139] Reynolds, G. (2010) Phys Ed: Can Exercise Moderate Anger? August 11, 2010. Available online, here: http://well.blogs.nytimes.com/2010/08/11/phys-ed-can-exercise-moderate-anger/?_r=0. Accessed: 16th June 2016.

[140] Byrne, J. (2018a) *Lifestyle Counselling and Coaching for the Whole Person: Or how to integrate nutritional insights, exercise and sleep coaching into talk therapy*. Hebden Bridge: The Institute for E-CENT Publications.

[141] Gordon, A.M. (2013) Up all night: the effects of sleep loss on mood. Research shows just one bad night of sleep can put a damper on your mood. *Psychology Today Online*. August 15th 2013. Available here: https://www.psychology today.com/ blog/ between-you-and-me/201308/all-night-the-effects-sleep-loss-mood. Accessed: 20th January 2018.

[142] MySahana (2012) Common Causes for Anger Management Issues. MySahana blog post. Online: http://mysahana.org/2012/02/common-causes-for-anger-manage-ment-issues/. Accessed: 22nd January 2018.

[143] Taylor-Byrne, R. (In press) Safeguard Your Sleep and Reap the Rewards: Better health, happiness and resilience. Hebden Bridge: The Institute for E-CENT Publications.

[144] Carroll, Helen, (2016) "How-losing-sleep-turn-women-MONSTERS-s-: It's known as sleep anger - or 'slanger'. And as these mothers confess, its toll on your family can be devastating", Daily Mail, Published: 23:15 13 January 2016 | Updated: 00:14, 14 January 2016.

http://www.dailymail.co.uk/femail/article-3398358/How-losing-sleep-turn-women-MONSTERS-s-known-sleep-anger-slanger-mothers-confess-toll-family-devastating.html#ixzz4xwxpvjlkDate accessed: 05/06/2018.

[145] The definition of the ***prefrontal cortex*** is that it is a part of the brain that lies at the very front of the brain, (just over your eyeballs) and it acts like the executive of a company, and manages complex processes such as reasoning things out, planning projects and goals for the future, using logic, memory, focussing attention, and blocking the expression of inappropriate or self-destructive impulses.

https://www.neuroscientificallychallenged.com/blog/2014/5/16/know-your-brain-prefrontal-cortex.

[146] Vitelli, Romeo,"Does Lack of Sleep make People More Violent"(2016) https://www.psychologytoday.com/gb/blog/media-spotlight/201610/does-lack-sleep-make-people-more-violent (date accessed 08/06/2018).

[147] Satir, V. (1972/1983) *Peoplemaking*. London: Souvenir Press. Chapter 5.

[148] Byrne, J.W. (2018b) *Top secrets for Building a Successful Relationship: Volume 1 – A blueprint and toolbox for couples and counsellors: C101*. Hebden Bridge: The Institute for E-CENT Publications.

[149] ".... Women are more likely to complain, criticize, or demand change during marital conflict, whereas men are more likely to avoid or withdraw; this gender disparity is one of the most reliable behavioural differences in the marital literature, particularly among distressed couples (Weiss & Heyman, 1990). Called the "wife demand-husband withdraw" or the "negative-withdraw" interaction sequence, it appears to be particularly destructive, linked both cross-sectionally and prospectively to marital discord (Christensen, 1987; Heavey, Lane, & Christensen, 1993). The gender differences in the negative-withdraw pattern have been explained in several ways. Christensen (1987) has argued that differences in the need for intimacy reflect, in part, divergent socialization experiences; in general, women want more closeness, whereas men seek more autonomy. Thus, wives demand and complain as a way of seeking intimacy, and husbands withdraw to maintain greater autonomy. Several studies have supported this conceptualization (Christensen, 1987; Christensen & Shenk, 1991). The conflict structure hypothesis relates gender differences in the negative-withdraw pattern to power differences in the structure of conflict (Heavey et al., 1993). For example, Jacobson (1983) has argued that traditional marital relationships provide greater benefits to men than women. Because men have less interest in changing the status quo, they are more likely to withdraw when confronted with their wives' requests for change. Data from two recent studies (Christensen & Heavey, 1990; Heavey et al., 1993) support this hypothesis." (Kiercolt-Glaser, 1996, page 325).

[150] For the Ohio State University research, "(the) researchers recruited 43 married couples, recording hostile behaviour and taking blood samples. Those who demonstrated more hostile behaviours had higher levels of one biomarker for leaky gut, and high levels of inflammation throughout the body". (Knapton, 2018).

[151] Bolton, R. (1979/1986). *People Skills: How to assert yourself, listen to others, and resolve conflicts.* Englewood Cliffs, NJ: Prentice-Hall Inc.

[152] Clinard, H.H. (1985) *Winning Ways to Succeed with People.* Houston: Gulf Publishing Company.

[153] Lindenfield, G. (2000) *Managing Anger: Simple steps to dealing with frustration and threat.* London: Thorsons.

[154] Sloane, W. (2010) *Anger Management: The essential guide.* Peterborough, UK: Need2Know/Forward Press Limited.

[155] Byrne, J. (2019) *Facing and Defeating your Emotional Dragons: How to process old traumas, and eliminate undigested pain from your past experience.* Hebden Bridge: The Institute for E-CENT Publications.

[156] Robinson, P. (2011) 'Could I send Mr Angry packing?' An article in the Femail section of the *Daily Mail Online.* 28th April 2011. Available online on this url: http://www.dailymail.co.uk/femail/article-1380989/Could-I-send-Mr-Angry-Packing-Horrified-repeatedly-raging-children-Philip-Robinson-tried-unconventional-therapy.html. Accessed: 6th June 2011.

[157] Fisher, M. (2005) *Beating Anger: The eight-point plan for coping with rage.* London: Rider.

[158] Robinson, P. (2011)

[159] Bernstein, B. (1960) Language and social class. *British Journal of Sociology, 11,* 271-276. And:

Bernstein, B. (1961) Social class and linguistic development: a theory of social learning. In: A.H. Halsey, J. Floud and L.A. Anderson (eds) *Education, Economy and Society.* Glencoe: Free Press. And:

Wood, D. (1988) *How Children Think and Learn.* Oxford: Blackwell. Pages 87-93.

[160] Byrne, J. (2011) Completing your experience of difficult events, perceptions and painful emotions. E-CENT Paper No.13. Hebden Bridge: The Institute for Emotive-Cognitive Embodied Narrative Therapy. Available online: https://ecent-institute.org/e-cent-articles-and-papers/

[161] Fisher, M. (2005) *Beating Anger: The eight-point plan for coping with rage.* London: Rider.

[162] Byrne, J. (2018) Lifestyle Counselling and Coaching for the Whole Person, as above.

[163] Pinker, S. (2015) *How the Mind Works.* London: Penguin Random House.

[164] Hobson, R.F. (1985) *Forms of Feeling: The heart of psychotherapy.* London: Routledge. Page 88.

[165] Paul Ekman (1993) identified the most universal, basic emotions - from a detailed international study - as: anger, fear, disgust, sadness, and enjoyment. See: Ekman, P. (1993) Facial expression and emotion. *American Psychologist 48 (4):* Pages 384-392.

[166] Turner, J.H. (2000) *On the Origins of Human Emotions. A sociological inquiry into the evolution of human affect.* Stanford University Press. See the book outline at this website: http://www.sup.org/ books/title/?id=436

[167] *The Dhammapada* (1973/2015) Taken from Juan Mascaró's translation and edition, first published in 1973. London: Penguin Books (Little Black Classics No.80)

[168] *The Dhammapada* (1973/2015)

[169] See page 245 of Cardwell, M. (2000) *The Complete A-Z Psychology Handbook.* Second edition. London: Hodder and Stoughton.

[170] Bretherton, I. (1992) The Origins of Attachment Theory: John Bowlby and Mary Ainsworth. *Developmental Psychology 28:* 759.

[171] Ayya Khema quotation taken from: Josh Baran (ed) (2003) *365 Nirvana: Here and now.* London: HarperCollins/Element.

[172] Epictetus (1991) *The Enchiridion.* New York: Prometheus Books.

[173] Aurelius, M. (1946/1992) *Meditations.* Trans. A.S.L. Farquharson. London: Everyman's Library.

[174] **First example**: 'Painkillers (are) behind most mass killings, say researchers' from a news item in the magazine, *What Doctors Don't Tell You*, dated August 2015, page 14. (This report is based on a published research study from the University of East Finland, published in *World Psychiatry, 2015; 14*:245-247). **Second example**: DrugWatch, an advocacy organization which supports people damaged by drugs, reports that people who take antidepressants: "...may experience side effects such as violent behavior, mania or aggression, which can all lead to suicide." Source: https://www.drugwatch .com/ssri/suicide/. And **Third example**: Patrick Holford has found evidence that brain allergies to particular foods and chemicals can cause emotional dysfunctions:

"The knowledge that allergy to foods and chemicals can adversely affect moods and behaviour in susceptible individuals has been known for a very long time. Early reports, as well as current research, have found that allergies can affect any system of the body, including the central nervous system. They can cause a diversity of symptoms including fatigue, slowed thought processes, irritability, agitation, aggressive behaviour, nervousness, anxiety, depression, schizophrenia, hyperactivity and varied learning disabilities." Source: http://www.alternativementalhealth.com/brain-allergieshow-sensitivities-to-food-and-other-substances-can-effect-the-mind/

[175] Darwin, C. (1872/1965) *The Expression of the Emotions in Man and Animals*. Chicago: University of Chicago Press.

[176] Evans, D. (2003) *Emotion: a very short introduction.* Oxford. Oxford University Press.

[177] Turner, J.H. (2000) *On the Origins of Human Emotions. A Sociological Inquiry into the Evolution of Human Affect*. Stanford University Press. See the book outline at: http://www.sup.org/books/title/?id=436

[178] *Sociality* is a measure of the extent to which individuals in an animal population tend to associate in social groups, and to form cooperative communities or societies.

[179] Panksepp, J. and Lucy Biven (2012) *The Archaeology of Mind: Neuroevolutionary Origins of Human Emotion*: W.W. Norton and Company. See the book description here: http://www.amazon.co.uk/The-Archaeology-Mind-Neuroevolutionary-Interpersonal/dp/0393705315

[180] Damasio, A. R. (1994). *Descartes' Error: emotion, reason and the human brain.* London, Picador.

[181] Siegel, D.J. (2015) *The Developing Mind: How relationships and the brain interact to shape who we are.* London: The Guilford Press.

[182] Byrne, J. (2009c) Rethinking the psychological models underpinning Rational Emotive Behaviour Therapy (REBT). E-CENT Paper No.1(a). Hebden Bridge: The Institute for E-CENT. Available online: https://ecent-institute.org/e-cent-articles-and-papers/

[183] Ellis, A. (1958). Rational Psychotherapy, *Journal of General Psychology,* 59, 35-49. And:

Ellis A. (1962). *Reason and Emotion in Psychotherapy,* New York, Carol Publishing.

[184] From a PowerPoint presentation by Jaak Panksepp, regarding his book: Panksepp, J. (1998) *Affective Neuroscience: The foundations of human and animal emotions.* Oxford University Press. Slide 12.

[185] LeDoux, J. (1996). *The Emotional Brain: the mysterious underpinnings of emotional life,* New York. Simon and Schuster.

[186] Mehrabian, A. (1981) *Silent messages: Implicit communication of emotions and attitudes.* Belmont, CA: Wadsworth (currently distributed by Albert Mehrabian, email: am@kaaj.com)

[187] Byrne, J. (2009b) The 'Individual' and his/her Social Relationships - The E-CENT Perspective. E-CENT Paper No.9. Hebden Bridge: The Institute for E-CENT. Available online: https://ecent-institute.org/e-cent-articles-and-papers/.

[188] Bowlby, J. (1988/2005) *A Secure Base.* London: Routledge Classics.

[189] Lewis, T., Amini, F. and Lannon, R. (2001) *A General Theory of Love.* New York: Vintage Books.

[190] Gerhardt, S. (2010) *Why Love Matters: How affection shapes a baby's brain.* London: Routledge.

[191] Siegel, D.J. (2015) *The Developing Mind: How relationships and the brain interact to shape who we are.* London: The Guilford Press.

[192] Hobson, R.F. (2000) *Forms of Feeling: the heart of psychotherapy.* London: Routledge.

[193] Panksepp, J. (1998) *Affective Neuroscience: The foundations of human and animal emotions.* Oxford University Press.

[194] Schore, A.N. (2015) *Affect Regulation and the Origin of the Self: The Neurobiology of Emotional Development.* London: Routledge.

[195] Smith, P.K., Cowie, H., and Blades, M. (2011) *Understanding Children's Development. Fifth edition.* Chichester, West Sussex: Wiley.

[196] Siegel, D.J. (2015) *The Developing Mind: How relationships and the brain interact to shape who we are.* London: The Guilford Press. Pages 152-153.

[197] Wallin, D.A. (2007) *Attachment in Psychotherapy.* New York: Guildford Press.

[198] Erwin, E. (1997) *Philosophy and Psychotherapy: Razing the troubles of the brain,* London, Sage.

~~~

www.ingramcontent.com/pod-product-compliance
Lightning Source LLC
Chambersburg PA
CBHW070321240526
45468CB00025B/1217